HOW TO DO IT

Volume 3

Published by the British Medical Journal
Tavistock Square, London WC1H 9JR

ISBN 0 7279 0269 5

Filmset by Eta Services (Typesetters) Ltd, Beccles, Suffolk
Printed in Great Britain by Latimer Trend & Company Ltd, Plymouth

With exams passed and qualifications gained, what more does a doctor need to know? All sorts of things, as the success of *How To Do It 1* and *How To Do It 2* showed. Now this third volume brings more expert advice to fill the gaps.

Contents

Organise a new department

S R NAIK

Organising a new department is not easy. This may be because there is no formal training in the art of organising departments except in the commercial or business arena. In this article I refer chiefly to problems governing the building and organisation of an academic medical department. Conventionally and sadly, the people who head these departments are selected by virtue of their seniority or sometimes their academic background rather than on their relevant qualifications and abilities for good organisation. Senior people often crave to occupy these positions because of the attendant power but they are often not aware of the responsibilities involved. Some of them may not even know that they are getting an opportunity to create something special.

It is true that very few senior people get an opportunity to start an altogether new department. Most simply move in as departmental heads when these positions are vacated. A few of my colleagues and I got a rare opportunity of moving from our positions as heads of established departments to organise brand new departments when our new institute of selected medical specialties opened about two years ago. All of us now agree that this has been a challenging although difficult job. But it has allowed us to build departments which could progress fast, free of rigid systems and narrow outlooks, which often limit the potential for improving or revamping established practices.

First thoughts

If you ever decide to take up the challenge of a new department I am sure you will subconsciously work out fresh ideas, strategies, and plans. The impressions formed of the departments you have worked in or visited in the past will be recalled. You will obviously want to have a first class department, one that will have few short-comings and most of the merits of the other departments. You will undoubtedly want to avoid the negative points of these depart-ments in your own; similarly, positive previous experiences will help you to entertain pleasant dreams for the future. From these images you can prepare a blueprint of your department, your own little brave new world.

Setting the goals

The first exercise you must undertake is deciding the goals of your department. There will always be some guidelines available; and yours may not be the first department of its kind. If it is going to be an academic medical department you will have to consider clinical services, training, and research as the three broad goals, but you will want to set your aims high and define the goals clearly and distinctively. How do you go about this? It is worth while at this stage to involve selected peers and like-minded professional colleagues, some of whom you could look forward to having with you as long term advisers and members of your staff. External ad-visers have a special importance because they can be forthright in their criticism and advice without being partisan. The key to the early steps in planning lies in drawing up this list of advisers who will give unflinching and genuine support to the department. It is of paramount importance to avoid choosing people whose motives are likely to clash with those of your department: it is better to have no one at all if that is the case.

As you proceed you will, of course, acquire your own initial staff members who should be handpicked and who should be thoroughly dependable and capable. Once you have acquired staff and advisers to help you, you must ensure, through a process of repeated dis-cussions and a fair exchange of views, that you all share broad aims and concepts in common. You are now in a position to propose a plan for the department. A thorough planning at this stage will in-clude outlining detailed plans of every section of the department and its functions. You will have to think in terms of reducing uncertainties to the minimum, bearing in mind that the overall plan will have to be tailored to suit budgets imposed by the institu-tion. .

Detailed proposal

After your proposal has been submitted, it will probably be scrutinised by the relevant body. Based on their comments and questions, you may be asked for further clarifications and justifications of some of the plans. If the plans are approved with or without modifications, you may be asked to make further detailed proposals. You may also have to give an expert opinion on issues that emerge from your special requirements. You may thus have to interact with different departments: (i) the stores department for technical equipment and consumables, (ii) furniture, stationery and pharmacy items, etc.; (iii) the architect for space requirement; (iv) the administrators for manpower; (v) the financial adviser for budgetary requirements.

Lucky are those whose needs are mundane enough to be covered by the standard manuals provided by the State or scientific societies. If you have planned for specialised and unusual functions about which these other departments have no clues whatsoever, you might have to sweat it out with your colleagues to prepare your demands in a stepwise manner. You should never omit the crucial step of consulting at this stage the persons who are ultimately going to do the actual work.

After all these discussions you will be in a position to present your demands under the following heads. Your department will have certain routine and specialised *functions*; these will be performed by different persons whose numbers, qualifications, and experience and other particulars you will project (*manpower*). All this planning will enable you to indicate where these people will physically be located (*space*) and which tools they will use (*equipment, etc*). You will calculate the costs of all the above demands as the initial capital cost, add to it the running or recurrent cost, and present an overall *budget proposal*.

Some of the points mentioned above require further discussion—namely, functions and manpower.

Functions

Detailing the functions of your department may be tricky, yet it is the most crucial and basic step on which all other requirements depend. Two aspects merit careful consideration before you decide on this vital issue.

3

(1) The first point is to decide if your department will perform specialised tasks based on certain "thrust area" programmes or whether it will be comprehensive in its functions. This may in turn depend on your area's particular needs—for example, if your centre is surrounded by several others which handle routine material there will be little point in your department doing the same. You should therefore carefully choose specific, well defined areas to provide newer facilities. The selection of thrust area programmes should be a conscious decision based on sound judgment. It is often prudent to limit and channel the development of the department and avoid haphazard growth.

(2) The second aspect of planning functions is that the department must be end-user stimulated. You may plan to investigate in depth patients with certain common diseases or you may want to launch selected treatment programmes. As a training organisation you need to keep in mind the requirements and aspirations of the trainee groups and how your training will help them to find useful employment. As a research unit you have to plan to find answers to selected questions which you have decided to look at. Undoubtedly this will be a dynamic area for which a flexible and adaptable approach will be invaluable.

Manpower planning

The department's manpower has to be planned carefully. In an academic medical department you plan for the faculty, technicians, and administrative staff. On the hospital side you will plan for nurses. There will be many other supporting staff members in other ranks that each section will need. You will have to exercise the utmost care to ensure that you have just the right number—no more or no less. Your detailed proposal for manpower will include a full complement, but you will fill the positions in phases. This will ensure that you allocate enough time for the adaptation and acclimatisation of the initial members so that a work ethic conforming to the values and aims of the department evolves smoothly.

With such scheduling you will learn more about the aptitudes, skills, strengths and the weaknesses of your existing staff and determine how they fit into your thrust programmes. An appraisal of the lacunae of the department at this stage will enable you to decide on the number and the type of new members to add to the team. At this stage you will also be in a better position to specify your requirements much more precisely than ever before.

While planning for skilled workers such as technicians or specialised nurses, it is unwise to assume that they will be freely available. It is therefore worth considering setting up your own training programme to make up the shortfall.

Choosing manpower

The task of finding the right kind of staff is indeed daunting, because although you will find around you bright and talented people, many of them may have adopted negative attitudes over the years and may have lost hope of realising their aspirations. You will therefore have to work slowly and cautiously to spot a combination of intelligence, talent, and optimism in your potential colleagues.

It is appropriate to discuss how best to select people who are most suited to carry out particular functions. Our present system is to advertise as widely as possible throughout the general and scientific press, detailing the type of person, the desired qualifications, experience, and aptitudes, and the salaries and benefits that can be offered. Details given are carefully honed to deter unnecessary applicants. Shortlisted candidates appear in front of a selection committee consisting of the head of our institution, the head of the department, and two or three of our listed advisers as experts. You could introduce variations in this process, depending on your needs and availability of candidates, set against the time frame of development of your department. For key positions I strongly recommend the practice of encouraging shortlisted candidates to visit your department before the interview. Many institutions in other countries offer positions to people on the basis of their past performance.

At the time of the interview itself the candidates and the head of the department must have adequate opportunities to talk with one another. As the head you must ensure the quality of the candidates and their suitability for the particular post. The candidates must be clear about what will be expected of them. If they have to opt to limit or change their sphere of work in terms of your thrust areas, this is the time to let them know. They must also know of salary and other benefits so that successful applicants are fully satisfied at the time of entry into the department.

5

The image of the department

Working atmosphere

The foundations of a successful department depend a lot on harmonious relationships and a measure of understanding among members; these help to build an early team spirit, which can be rather difficult to inculcate later on in the day.

You might be amused to know how many trivial matters determine departmental harmony and standing. Take the example of a new member—a staff member or a trainee entering your department. He or she comes in with some apprehension, hope, or even awe. He or she naturally expects a certain type of reception such as a warm greeting, friendly introduction to other members, familiarisation with the new surroundings, and finally certain practical facilities like a desk, a chair etc. I know of people who have resigned soon after joining because some of these conditions had not been met. On the other hand, if you are exuberant in your reception of a new member, older members may view it somewhat jealously. These are situations which you will have to face with some knowledge of human psychology.

You will have to provide a sense of security and self esteem for all your team members through education, consultation, appreciation and other incentives. Your team member must be made to feel valuable and useful to the department to encourage a sense of belonging and pride. There will be tussles and frictions among individuals and demands for more facilities, so much so that you will find it difficult to distinguish between need and greed. But you will have to ensure that these problems are solved in such a way that the department emerges as a fair, just, and decent place in which to work. Opportunities for meeting informally at this stage are also an important means of creating an atmosphere of cordiality, friendliness, and openness. Your team members are the department's best ambassadors.

Public relations

Does a department need ambassadors? Whatever the debate on the issue, the answer is that you cannot function in isolation. The department shares with the institution the responsibility of service to the public and end-users. The watchdogs of the institution's performance include the media, voluntary groups, and end-users. To an academic medical department the end-users may be patients, students, research workers and others, who look forward to being members of your department. Points of contact with these groups and individuals must therefore be smooth and gentle. There could be many examples of these contact points—patients attending a busy outpatient clinic, students appearing at an entrance examination, or candidates facing a job interview. All these people will have variable perceptions of the likely treatment they will receive in your department. Anticipating and understanding them will enable you to provide fair and decent treatment. You must, however, ensure that these attempts at public relations are spontaneous and not contrived.

Myths and slogans

Public relations, and in equal measure, interpersonal relationships within the department, should be not based on myths and slogans about the policies of the department. Minor successes often prompt departmental heads to publicise vociferously their policies. Other heads project themselves as moral models for other members to emulate. Such actions are, to say the least, short sighted and harmful to the department in the long term. They impose heavy demands on all the members to live up to the propaganda and distract them from their real duties. It is therefore far better to keep a low profile and maintain a genuine and sincere devotion to the main activities of the department. Allow your department to be seen as human, accessible, and even vulnerable rather than mechanical, snobbish, and overefficient.

Running a new department

You will find running a new department an altogether different ball game if you have so far been looking after an established unit. Your leadership qualities will be tested as never before. You and your colleagues will be under a constant strain to develop continuously the department, and you will be watched within and outside it with expectations, hope, and cynicism. The demands to perform more, quicker, and better will lead to clashes of interest and a lot of mental tension for all concerned.

A particularly important issue is that of providing promotional avenues to people at the right moment. Stagnation of people who perform well is an early sign of malfunction of the department. If your members have to come and ask you for promotions, it could be humiliating for them and undermine your role as leader. There may also be a difficult case of an obviously poor performer who entered the department in spite of your careful selection process. He or she will need educating, motivating, and if these do not work, relocating and even weeding out as tactfully as possible. Harnessing and channelling the energies and talents of your gifted members and making use of others' obviously limited qualities are crucial to steering your department through these rough days towards its declared goals.

Monitoring progress

Once you have built your department, you have to sustain its progress. You will almost certainly need to introduce at this stage some way of obtaining feedback on your performance. Your end-users—patients, trainees, volunteers for clinical research—as well as your team members, peers, and advisers can all give you help. Have all these people been asked for their views? Are they satisfied that your department has performed well and met its goals?

The simplest way to start this type of monitoring is to keep registers for complaints, comments, and suggestions at several convenient points for your end-users and encourage them to enter their views, anonymously if they prefer. The feedback must be collated and discussed in your departmental meetings and adequate steps to redress grievances or improve an existing service should be set in motion.

When you review the points entered in your feedback register you might be able to design "proformas" to structure these inputs, in a way which makes it easier for the end-user to give his or her views and which will give you adequate guidance for future improvements.

Conclusions

Organising a department is a difficult exercise, but it is possible to achieve your goals and feel proud of your creation. During the exercise, you will hopefully have learnt of your capabilities and equally of your failings and will have devised your own ways of enlisting help in areas where you are likely to fail. You will thus have built a human and not a mechanical organisation.

You will perhaps also have come to realise that there are better people than you to handle several aspects of your organisation, to some of whom you can hand over the organisation eventually. For there will come a time when you will want to do this. When you do, look back with satisfaction on what you have created, know that it is something good, but that the best is yet to come there or elsewhere.

Suggested reading

Bryman A. *Leadership and organization*. London: Routledge and Kegan Paul, 1986.
Cutlip S M, Center A H. *Effective public relations* 5th ed. New York: Prentice-Hall Inc, 1978.
Stewart V, Stewart A. *Managing the poor performer*. London: Gower Publishing Co Ltd, 1988.

Write a job description

R FIRTH

A job description is probably one of the most neglected and under-rated documents in employment. When they do exist job descriptions are often poorly written and out of date. In many instances they are non-existent—strange treatment for such an important document which, if used properly, should represent the essential foundations on which employer and employee relations are built.

Importance of the job description

Recruitment and selection of staff—At the outset of the recruitment and selection process it is important to have an accurate and up to date job description. This gives the recruiter, who is often not directly concerned or familiar with the particular post, an appreciation of the duties and responsibilities of the job and helps in deciding on the most appropriate method of recruitment, advertising media, and interview techniques and, finally, in considering the suitability of the applicants. A job description is also useful for the applicants, giving them a better appreciation of the extent of the job.

Job grading—Any system of job grading, whether formal or informal, relies heavily on the existence of job descriptions, which often provide the most effective means of understanding the extent of duties and the relative values of various jobs within an organisation.

Appraisal of performance—In its simplest form an appraisal of performance aims at assessing performance against the agreed duties of the job. Absence of a detailed job description can lead to misunderstandings and uncertainties, which often contribute to poor performance.

Training—In the development of a structured training programme the job description provides a useful starting point in establishing the skills and knowledge required to complete the tasks of the job satisfactorily, and this in turn should help to highlight individual training needs.

Supervisor–staff relations—Often a breakdown in relations can be traced to a lack of understanding of or disagreement about the extent of the duties and responsibilities of a post—a problem that is usually overcome or avoided by the existence of a detailed job description.

Content and format

There is no set approach for writing a job description that is suitable for all jobs, and generally a more senior and complex job requires a more detailed job description than a junior and fairly simple job. As a general rule aim at keeping it as brief as possible. Usually only the main duties and responsibilities would be included.

Although the format varies considerably, most job descriptions cover certain main areas. (1) Personal and organisational information is given—including the job title, the location of the job and the department, the title of the person to whom the employee reports, and the name of the person who prepared the job description and the date of its completion. If appropriate the number of people reporting to the employee should be mentioned. In many organisations the name of the current job holder would also be included. (2) A brief statement—usually restricted to one or at most two sentences—encapsulates the main purpose of the job. (3) For senior management posts the description usually includes some of the main dimensions associated with the job—for example, the number of people employed, the size of revenue, the turnover, and the capital controlled. (4) The main section of the description identifies the main duties of the job—usually as a detailed list of duties or in narrative form—in both cases the aim is to specify clearly the main tasks. (5) Many descriptions also include details of the qualifications and level of education, experience, and skills appropriate to the job. Although this is more of a "person specification" than a description of the job, it nevertheless fits quite comfortably within a job description as it helps in forming an overall impression of the job. There is an increasing tendency to include details of certain terms and conditions of employment—for example, hours of work,

---

ABC Corporation

Job description

Job Title: Secretary

Department: Finance

Relationships:
   (*a*) Immediate supervisor: head of department
   (*b*) Subordinates directly supervised: none
   (*c*) Other persons with whom you have regular working contact:
       all members of Finance Department. Limited contact with
       members of other departments. Telephone contact with
       suppliers

Main purpose of the job:
   To provide secretarial support to the head of department

Main duties and responsibilities:
   (*a*) Typing of correspondence, memos, and reports
   (*b*) Keeping diary, arranging meetings, and organising travel
   (*c*) Maintaining filing and bring forward systems

Education and training and experience required:
   "O" level English and Maths minimum
   Secretarial training and secretarial experience at a senior level
   Confident shorthand—90 words per minute or more (used
   recently). Word processing skills preferred

October 1987

---

rates of pay, on call arrangements, but unless the case for doing
otherwise is particularly strong, this type of information should
more properly be left to the contract of employment. (6) In large
complex organisations it is often advisable to attach a copy of the
departmental or divisional organisation chart as an aid to clarifying
precisely where the job fits into the organisation.

Who writes job descriptions

There are several options as to who should write a job description, and the determining factor is usually the size and structure of
the organisation. A job description may be written by the current
employee, by his or her manager or jointly, by a specialist job
analyst, or, in some cases, a committee.

XYZ Institute

Job description

Job title: Librarian   *Location:* London

Department: Central library

Principal purpose of job:
To lead the development of information services in the institute's library

Staff supervised:
Library services manager, three assistant librarians

Responsibility for equipment:
Extensive microcomputing equipment, including DEC Micro Vax 2000, IBM and BBC microcomputers, CDROM mass storage device, optical character reader, photocopiers, and other office equipment

Financial responsibilities:
Yearly budget in excess of £250 000
Capital equipment and library stock (nominal) £800 000

Main duties:
Planning and implementation of policies to provide cost effective library services
Liaison with librarians of other national and international university and professional libraries to develop strategies of library services
Initiation and management of new information storage and retrieval projects
Planning and implementing library routines to achieve optimum utilisation of stock for the benefit of members
Representing the institute at national and international meetings on librarianship and information science
Statutory duty (under copyright legislation) to recover costs of providing photocopies; setting up a computer invoicing system to ensure recovery of money owed
Responsibility for the storage, use, preservation, and refurbishment of old and valuable library books

Education, training, and experience
Degree or postgraduate diploma in librarianship or information science
Fellow or associate of the Library Association or equivalent qualification
Proved ability to initiate and manage information science projects

Prepared by: ....   Date ....

The employee should have a better understanding of the job than anybody else and should therefore be well placed to write the job description. There are, however, several possible pitfalls—the employee may for instance be too subjective or may not be doing the job correctly, when the resultant description is probably inaccurate. Although the manager should have the advantage of having an overall view of the job, this may not be sufficiently detailed to do justice to a detailed job description. The joint approach is probably the most effective, the employee preparing a first draft which is vetted and eventually approved by the manager, through a process of open discussion. Of course, in the case of a new job this option would not be available. Larger organisations often employ specialist job analysts, some of whose duties are to write job descriptions. This approach has some obvious advantages, such as consistency, impartiality, and experience, but substantial input by the employee and his or her manager and the authority of the manager for final approval are still advisable. Although rather uncommon, in some organisations job descriptions are written and approved by a committee. This can be cumbersome and should be avoided when possible.

Whatever the system maximum uniformity of format, terminology, and the amount of detail is important, particularly when job descriptions are used to evaluate jobs or for grading, when there is a danger that the length of the job description will influence its rating. Also the job description is intended to describe the job—not the person doing it.

When to write job descriptions

Ideally, a job description should be completed before the job is filled, but this may not always be possible in a business that is introducing a system of providing job descriptions. In this case the right time is "as soon as is practicable"—having first cleared the necessary staff communications and agreed the system and method to be adopted. One word of caution, however—starting and maintaining an effective system of job descriptions is not easy and requires much effort and a disciplined approach. The potential pay off, however—in terms of greater efficiency, better quality of recruitment and selection, greater job satisfaction, and improved staff relations—makes the investment well worth while.

Writing job descriptions

- Decide on the system best suited to your business
- Ensure appropriate communication with staff concerned
- Aim at consistency
- Ensure maximum involvement of current employee
- Keep descriptions as brief as possible
- Ensure effective maintenance and updating of relevant records.

Appoint a colleague

M C PETCH

Appointing a colleague is rather like choosing a spouse, except that divorce is not really an option. In both cases you have to live with the consequences of your decision for several decades and you may mistakenly believe that you are in control, whereas in reality there is usually some mother in law like figure manipulating events. Do not be alarmed by this. Arranged marriages can be most successful because neither party has undue expectations of the other. Provided you can live with the other party the marriage can be made to work and your differences will lead to a stronger unit. My experience of seeing the NHS consultant appointments system in action may help show others how to, or not to, choose a colleague.

These comments apply only to senior NHS appointments. Academic posts should be subject to more liberal rules.

Preliminaries

The preliminaries take a long time, often a year or more in the case of a vacancy due to retirement. As soon as a close colleague whispers his or her intention of going start planning. Decide what you want to do because at this stage a short friendly discussion will enable you to take over the desirable parts of your colleague's practice and shed, or at least share, the undesirable parts of yours. Then write down carefully the sessional commitments that must be covered. For a cardiologist this might include two or more clinics, two investigative sessions, three ward rounds, one or two sessions in coronary care, two for administration, one for reading and research, one for teaching, one for travel; already the week is overbooked. It might seem obvious to you that there is a pressing need for a replacement but do not be surprised when this is challenged. Write down why a replacement is essential and take this

NHS consultant committee is made up of:

- Lay chairman appointed by regional health authority
- District representatives:
  (a) lay member of the health authority
  (b) specialist medical representative
- Medical representatives of:
  (a) appropriate college
  (b) region concerned (two)
  (c) university

and your provisional job description to the district medical officer, whose advice should be sought early and in confidence. When your retiring colleague begins to talk about dates the news will already be widespread, and urgent claims for new consultants in other disciplines will be presented from the most surprising quarters. Be prepared.

The details of the job description have to be discussed by the medical advisory committee of the relevant district hospital, often a consultant staff council. Make sure your friends are there; you may find that you don't have many on the day. If the chairman at least understands your case you may get your job description accepted with minor modifications. If the chairman does not then the matter will be deferred for a month, and then another month, and so on. If two districts are concerned your task is at least doubled. Eventually a job description must be agreed even though your secretary can spot the flaws. Keep a careful record of these discussions. Many months may yet elapse before the appointment, and during these months people will forget that they ever took place. They may assert later that they did not have the opportunity for comment. To avoid this it is important to ensure that all potentially interested parties see a copy of the job description.

At this stage you will also become aware that the senior registrar grapevine is waiting for the advertisement. At meetings colleagues you hardly know will explain that their own time expired senior registrar is very good and thoroughly worthy of "your" job. Listen politely and question discreetly. Treasure the comments because as the time of the appointment draws near colleagues will become more elaborate with the truth. Information volunteered casually at

---

*To see all applicants is time
consuming ...
To see some seems unjust. To see
none is a luxury that only
uninvolved
members can afford ...
But all serious candidates should be
seen.*

---

a conference dinner is likely to be more accurate than that elicited
by direct questioning once the shortlist has been made.

The advertisement

A short conventional advertisement in the *BMJ* is sufficient.
Health authorities that take several column inches merely an-
nounce their fear that there may be few applicants. If the job is
unattractive then you should have recognised this and taken steps
to improve it beforehand. In cardiology, for example, there is a
lack of suitably trained senior registrars for consultant posts in district hospitals. A simple and mutually beneficial arrangement may
be to link such posts with a regional centre giving opportunities for
cardiac catheterisation, for instance. There are other similar
devices to improve a job.

The timing of the advertisement should allow for the following:
one month or so before the closing date, a further month for shortlisting (before and during these months an appointments committee will be chosen and a date for the appointment agreed,
although this may take longer if one potential member is important
and busy), two weeks for the appointment to be confirmed, and
then three months for the successful candidate to work out his or
her notice. Six months therefore elapse between the appearance of
the advertisement and the provision of a service. An interregnum is
unsatisfactory but has unsuspected advantages—desks are cleared,
clinics dwindle, a locum may shed light on your former colleague's
habits, and of course the regional health authority may save
money.

Trawling for applicants is generally a mistake. A potential
applicant who is working overseas may merit a letter and a copy of

the job description, but more active canvassing may secure an applicant who is successful and later decides not to take up the appointment or does so only to leave shortly afterwards.

Appointments committee

NHS consultant appointment committees are statutorily constituted and are empowered to make a recommendation to the regional health authority, which invariably ratifies the recommendation. The members of the committee must be: a lay chairman (appointed by the regional health authority); district representatives: lay member of the health authority, specialist medical representative; medical representatives of the appropriate (*a*) college, (*b*) region—two, one of whom, a non-specialist medical representative, is often selected by the district, (*c*) university.

There are variations on this basic theme. For example, if two districts are concerned then an extra member is allowed, or if an unrepresented department feels particularly aggrieved it may be represented by an observer. All appears to be straightforward and democratic.

But who appoints the appointments committee? This is largely mysterious. The flavour of the committee of course determines the recommendation. Hence the choice of committee members is vitally important. It is difficult, however, to escape the conclusion that powerful and undemocratic forces are often at work. At district level the members are chosen by the consultant staff council. This is, of course, perfectly fair provided that they choose you. It might be thought that a regional medical advisory committee would choose the regional medical representative and that a body such as the cardiology committee of the Royal College of Physicians might choose the college representative. But no. The choice appears to be arrived at by a process of consultation that is difficult to fathom. When the behaviour of a member of an appointments committee is bizarre there is no redress. This aspect of the appointments system needs reform.

The members of an appointments committee are responsible for drawing up the shortlist. Most members will make up their list from the submitted applications with no personal knowledge of the candidates. Those members who are going to have to work very closely with the successful applicant need to do more. To see all applicants is very time consuming and may be impossible. To see

---

*Only those applicants whom you
can work with over a decade or
more and who have the necessary
qualifications should be shortlisted.*

---

some seems unjust. To see none is a luxury that only uninvolved members can afford. There is no easy compromise, but all serious candidates should be seen.

Some candidates are exemplary in their organisation. They arrange a visit to suit your convenience, turn up on time, ask a few relevant questions, see the department, say thank you, and express a wish to come back if they are shortlisted. Others just make difficulties: they will trip you up in conversation, criticise your department to others, ask if the job description can be altered, and may even lodge a complaint against you—all of which are memorable recent experiences. Usually there are too many of the first group. Your responsibility is to try to treat them all equally, even though you know that you can work better with some.

An NHS consultant is appointed to provide a service in a particular discipline. Unfortunately, this is the one talent that cannot be assessed at an appointments committee. Undue weight is invariably given to a candidate's research publications. His or her capacity for continued service has to be gauged from informal consultation before the interview. The chief fault with the present system of appointing consultants is the lack of opportunity for assessing a candidate's clinical ability and the likelihood that he or she will continue to provide a service over two decades in the face of such temptations as private practice, etc. Hence the importance of previous informal consultations.

Any curriculum vitae will naturally look splendid. Publications will be there in plenty. But no one will tell you whether these were acquired by evening and weekend work or by delegating clinical duties to registrars and senior house officers. There is a strong case for allowing candidates to list only a few publications, perhaps three presentations, three original papers, and a review article or a book. References from senior medical staff, which are generally presented at the time of the interview, are likewise paeons of praise. What you really need to do is to have a word with an outpatient sister, ward clerk, or medical secretary—namely, someone who can tell you whether a candidate pulls his weight. The vast majority do of course; hence such testimonials are regarded as superfluous. There seems to be no good reason why the performance of senior registrars should be judged solely by their seniors; they may be at their best when their seniors are away. Perhaps in future a shorter CV should be balanced by more testimonials including, perhaps, a nurse's, an administrator's, or a junior doctor's.

The length of the shortlist is an easy matter; six is too many. Only those applicants whom you can work with over a decade or more and who have the necessary qualifications should be shortlisted.

Shortlisted candidates will usually pay several visits and will generally be invited to attend a "trial by sherry" on the evening before the interview. This dyspeptic experience gives everyone a chance to meet their potential colleague. We asked our unit administrator along; you should do likewise. Let the district medical officer be master of ceremonies, he will find it easier to get rid of the guests and can supervise the subsequent discussion while you make notes and watch your present colleagues empty the bottles.

The interview

Everything truly hinges on the interview. Whatever machinations have taken place beforehand are now exposed. The power blocs become apparent. You can only watch with fascination as experienced committee members have their way. You may wish that you had taken more trouble to influence people before, yet to have done so may have laid you open to the charge of trying to fix the job.

There is in practice little opportunity for detailed questioning. If five candidates are shortlisted and if each member spends only five minutes talking to the candidate and an additional five minutes are allowed for changeover then the interview will last three hours, and that is before any discussion can take place.

These three hours may be a revelation. The candidate that you thought was ideally qualified for the job may be destroyed by subtle questioning. Another may reveal an inadequate understanding of the job despite your careful explanation and job description. A third may admit to liking clinical work but goes home at 6 00 pm to help put the children to bed instead of pursuing laboratory research. The strengths and weaknesses of the committee system are exposed in this most crucial of all committees. The tension is inevitable because so much is at stake and because you and the other medical members will remember the day when your own future career was being assessed in a similar fashion. Unlike every other medical committee, no one nods off.

The order of interviewing and speaking is generally the same; the college representative speaks first, then those least concerned with the job, and finally the district representatives including yourself. Usually, and perhaps surprisingly, the decision is immediate and unanimous. Rarely is no appointment made, the usual reason being that the job is in some way deficient. The fact that so many appointments turn out to be a success may have more to do with earlier selection than the final consultant interview. Senior registrars are a select group of highly talented, industrious, agreeable, and strongly motivated people.

You do not have to ask questions; you will probably have asked all the important ones beforehand. You may wish to ask one or two to clear up any confusion created by other members. Remarkably, other members may be offensive about your department; if you can rise above the temptation to criticise theirs then you will be proud of yourself afterwards.

Afterwards

You will not know whether you have made the correct choice until at least two, and probably five, years have elapsed, but two things you will know. Firstly, you will feel that there has to be a better method of appointing a colleague. And secondly, you are no longer viewed as the new, energetic, young consultant. Suddenly polite colleagues are describing you as the doyen of the service, while most think of you as quaintly senile.

Choose a house officer

JOHN S YUDKIN

As with much else in health care in Britain market forces have a major effect on the process of choosing a house officer. The professorial house surgeon job, or a senior house officer rotation in medicine at a district general hospital with a good membership course, is probably going to be more oversubscribed than a psychogeriatric post in Rejkyavik. If you are in the seller's market it can be quite an ego trip to find so many bright eyed young people falling over themselves to work for you, even though this is a bit like taking pleasure at being at a slave market. But how do you decide who is the best candidate for the job?

The selection of candidates for a medical job requires receipt of a curriculum vitae plus interview, a process which has changed little in living memory. Why the medical profession should have been left standing at the lights, while industry has zoomed off over the horizon, may reflect the innate conservatism of our profession. On the other hand, it seems that the method works reasonably well, and in general the two parties seem to end up viewing the process as reasonably fair (except for those who don't get appointed). This interpretation probably reflects a general unwillingness to dip toes into new and uncharted waters. But you will need to ensure that your selection process is fair, and, increasingly, seen to be so.

What are you looking for?

Different consultants have diverse views about what qualities they want in a house officer. Some are determined to select someone in their own image, a process of cloning which antedated by some years the discovery of reverse transcriptase, and which is helped by the fact that the newly qualified doctor has often acquired many of the attitudes and prejudices of his or her teachers, albeit with a more limited transfer of knowledge and skills. Despite my critical tone, I think the habit may be widespread; my present juniors have heard themselves described as radical extremists during the campaign about junior doctors' hours of duty.

The requirements which would be fairly universally accepted, besides a level of knowledge and skill which would make the person competent to perform the routine tasks of every day practice, are the following abilities:

   (i) to act in emergency situations in an organised manner;
  (ii) to know when to ask for help;
 (iii) to relate sympathetically to patients, even when pushed or tired;
 (iv) to work well with other members of the firm, other health workers, and students;
  (v) to organise the workload, both to facilitate patient care and to permit adequate time for relaxation;
 (vi) to learn from observation, advice, and experience, and adapt accordingly;
(vii) to contribute to informed debate, without uncritical acceptance of all dogma.

In essence what you are probably looking for is someone in whom you would happily place your patients' care when you aren't there.

Many of these characteristics are impossible to judge in any way other than by working with the person for the duration of a six month job. It is, of course, possible that you will have worked with the applicant before, perhaps as a medical student or locum attached to your firm, or in a more junior post in the same hospital, and if so, this simplifies the selection process. The two house physicians I have most liked and respected were both on my firm for their first clinical student attachment, and with each of them it was apparent from the first few days that they would be the sort of doctors in whose hands I would happily put myself if I were ill. Nevertheless, there are many hazards in relying on personal preference, rather than on judgment of skills and abilities, in selecting your house officer.

The selection process

The process of choosing a house officer is open to bias and prejudice. It is, happily, no longer acceptable or legal to discriminate on the grounds of gender or race, but doubtless there are still examples of such discrimination in action. Your district is likely to have an equal opportunities policy and you may well find yourself contravening this if you are not careful to keep personal prejudice out of the selection process. Many health authorities offer training in selection and interviewing processes and in equal opportunities awareness. Guidelines for selecting, shortlisting, and interviewing include producing an agreed job description, writing specifications of the qualities applicants require for the post, and keeping careful notes on the grounds whereby candidates are excluded, as these would be necessary in any claims against the authority which went to industrial tribunal. This is another area of the selection process in which the medical profession has some catching up to do, but it clearly can no longer consider itself either beyond reproach or beyond recrimination.

The curriculum vitae

If you have a much larger number of applicants than there are posts available you will have to whittle the numbers down to a short list. In general, the application form and curriculum vitae are the first pieces of information you will have about your potential house officer. Candidates surely realise that they can make or break themselves by their application, so it is surprising that the quality of these documents is so variable.

You can learn a great deal about someone's character and suitability for a post by reading a covering letter explaining why they feel that this job is right for them, or a curriculum vitae which gives more than the crudest chronological details of education and previous posts. The quality of the document is also important. The poorly photocopied curriculum vitae, with the last three posts added in handwriting with different inks, gives a poorer impression than one produced on the applicant's Amstrad—and it may be valuable to know that one's potential house officer is computer literate. And talking of literacy, I suspect it is not just my own personal fetish to prefer house officers who can spell.

The content of the curriculum vitae may also be useful. I don't feel that a previous PhD, a BSc, or a list of publications is that important in the selection process at house officer level, where the main function of the job is involvement in patient care. The performance of clinical tasks and the acquisition of knowledge and skills do not seem to correlate well with academic qualifications, and I even have my doubts that the scientific content of BSc courses really instils a more scientific or critical approach in the graduates. Nor, it seems, does the huge variety of experiments across the country in innovative approaches to medical education translate into doctors easily identified as, say, "obviously a Southampton graduate" or "a Bart's chap". The range of characteristics of newly qualified doctors is so wide that any small difference attributable to the medical school would be missed as a type II error, and in any event is more likely a result of differences in admission policy rather than in the course itself. Nevertheless, there may be something on the curriculum vitae, like the medical school, or a hockey blue, or an Arsenal supporter, that you decide is grounds enough for offering the job.

The curriculum vitae should be used to get some view of the applicant's character, and not just to decide that the person should be capable of performing the tasks required. The description of the elective period, of holiday jobs or work experience before medical school, of participation in a student psychotherapy scheme, or of leisure time activity will give a more rounded impression. It is, however, quite difficult to know how to react to statements like: "my most important personal influences have been Nietzsche and Charlie Parker".

The interview

Although the process of selection by interview has its critics, I feel that it is a valuable way of seeing how you will relate to your potential house officer. There are candidates who are struck mute, or who are clearly terrified by the whole occasion, while others are so laid back about it that they may seem to be trying to put the interview panel at their ease. Although on occasions the former is merely the result of panic at the sight of the panel of 12 senior professionals across a table, or the latter a manifestation of β-blockade, it is my view that the impression given at interview is often the factor which, given that any of the short listed applicants could probably do the job well, best differentiates the one person with whom you will most enjoy working from the rest.

In many walks of life the standard interview format is being replaced as the sole selection method, and you may decide that—for example, you would like, in addition or instead, to invite all your short listed candidates to spend a half day attached to your firm. The structure of junior hospital jobs, however, may make this difficult to arrange. Another possible constraint is that you may not be selecting house officers as an individual, but as part of a linked house job scheme, or for a postgraduate training scheme for all senior house officer posts in the hospital, which may impose limits on what is feasible. You may want to see applicants yourself before the interview, ostensibly to let them have a look around and find out about the job, but really to provide the opportunity for a one-to-one discussion. For the selection process itself, even if it is for just your job, it is important not to interview on your own. Another consultant or your registrar can be a useful contributor to help balance bias, and the hospital personnel department may wish to be involved. Even if you don't see them before the interview, it is important to encourage candidates to come to the hospital to have a look around, and if someone else shows them the ropes, and not their potential consultant, the risk of bias can be reduced. The candidate who has seen the hospital and who has spoken to the present house officers is clearly interested in the job.

Interviews can be very boring—for both sides of the table. To sit through a series of 15 sets of "why do you want to come and work here?" is unlikely to give much insight into personality. On the other hand, an equal opportunities policy means that you should cover the same broad area with each candidate. It is certainly not acceptable, for example, to ask only female applicants what are their plans for a family. In selecting topics it is worth picking up interesting items from the curriculum vitae, quite aside from obvious plants like Nietzsche and Charlie Parker. You will be able to get a good idea of how well the applicants can think on their feet by asking rather less obvious questions—such as, "what lessons for the organisations of health care in the United Kingdom did you learn from your elective in the Amazon Basin?" You will certainly find interviews more interesting and the responses more varied if you introduce topics such as ethics, or prevention, or health care structure into the interview. For example, you could experiment by asking the candidates how they might cope with a described case in which there is a conflict of interest about confidentiality, or what they think about the concept of GPs' use of deputising services in the light of campaigns about hours of work. If you are confident in your skills in the performing arts you might even attempt a five minute role play, although the pale, sweaty, un-β-blocked candidate is likely to be turned into a jibbering wreck by this approach.

The references

At pre-registration level you will probably have references from the sub-dean of the medical school, and perhaps a consultant for whom the applicant did a student assistantship, but these are unlikely to provide much more insight to character than would a bank manager's reference, and merely attest to medical solvency. At the senior house officer level a telephone call from one of the referees may be more informative than words on paper. Phrases like "the best houseman I have ever had" or "a high flyer" abound, but you occasionally still see references like the apocryphal, "Dr X has performed his tasks entirely to his own satisfaction". Many referees are keener to tell you what a good, or busy, job they provide. Others may give you good material for between-the-lines detective work—such phrases as "she has matured in approach during the tenure of this post", or "with supervision, his clinical skills are reasonably safe", may give cause for concern.

Allocating people to jobs

If you are interviewing on your own your first choice will usually be your next house officer. If, however, you are part of a linked house officer scheme your preference list may be subjected to a process of computer matching. It is remarkable how much acrimony this seemingly objective process arouses, with paranoia in the district general hospital that some three-to-one matches are more equal than other one-to-one matches (especially if the former is on the professorial unit). It is, however, equally likely that dissatisfaction will ensue from the computerless panel interview. In our district the senior house officer interviews, which take place every six months, produce a surprising degree of consensus on who should be appointed, but with much cattle trading on who gets allocated to which job. You might discuss with your colleagues approaches such as rotating the option of first choice, for example to the short-listers, or, unless you are the most junior, giving the senior consultant first option. It should be possible for the candidates and the consultants all to write down their first three choices and to attempt a point scoring system, but the matching process may take a very long time without a computer.

Conclusion

When I was asked by the editor to share my expertise in this area, I felt that it would be far easier to write a *How To Do It* on something where the correct performance of the task could be readily evaluated. I would be happier, for example, writing about how to give insulin—but perhaps choosing a house officer needn't be so different. Except that in the former case you'd use a needle, not a pin.

Be a manager

CYRIL CHANTLER

There is no right or wrong way to learn how to be a manager, and in this respect management is quite different from medicine or science. My qualification for being asked to write this article is that I have spent three years as chairman of our hospital board of management, with the title of unit general manager but without any specific training apart from reading a book while on a long journey before taking up my appointment.[1] I have read two other books since[2,3]; Sir John Harvey Jones's *Making it Happen* I recommend to any clinician or academic because it emphasises the importance of leadership with its characteristics of imagination, courage, and sensitivity. Management is not the same as command or administration, but it requires characteristics derived from both. I am concerned mostly with the contribution that clinicians can make to the success of the NHS.

Qualifications

Many doctors have management experience, though they commonly discount this and spend little time analysing it. Most will have been required to organise activities on behalf of others at school, at university, or in practice. They are also experienced at making difficult decisions with inadequate information. They learn to live with the consequences while being prepared to accept that when they are wrong they must try again, driven by their responsibility for other people's lives and health. Sometimes they find it difficult to accept that management, like medicine, is an inexact science. At least as far as hospitals are concerned, management is as important as medicine because doctors can serve their patients only if the resources are available and the whole team is organised to work at maximum efficiency.

30

Clinicians are natural leaders in a hospital. They, more than any other group, make the decisions that most affect the activities of the whole organisation. Consultants are usually associated intimately with a single hospital over many years. They are well educated and intelligent (intelligence being a necessary criterion for entry to the profession) and undoubtedly develop stamina in the early years after qualification. A sense of humour, if not natural, is certainly a common defence against the tensions of the job. All of these characteristics are useful for a manager. Doctors and managers ought to be good listeners: attentive listening is essential for obtaining a clinical history from a patient, which enables the nature of a problem to be defined clearly in a relatively brief time. Doctors concerned with management are, surprisingly, not always as skilled as might be expected at counselling staff and making decisions that may affect employees profoundly. Sometimes a natural loyalty to people hampers decisions that are vital to the hospital. It is no use keeping people in jobs that are not necessary or in which their performance is poor; it is far better to help them by analysing their performance, providing motivation, retraining them, or occasionally allowing them to leave with proper entitlements.

Strategy and structure

It is always worth spending a great deal of time thinking and talking about the strategy of the organisation and making sure the structure is, or remains, correct. In 1984 Guy's Hospital was faced with a reduction in its budget of nearly 20% over eight years. The previous five years had been characterised by closures of beds, inadequate replacement of equipment, little expenditure on the infrastructure of the hospital, and falling morale with increasing antagonism between different professional groups. Consultant staff, angered by their inability to provide care and by problems ranging from lengthening waiting lists to the frequent absence of outpatients' records, made formal representations at all levels of the health service, and many of us took advantage of the proximity of Guy's Hospital to Fleet Street and the media to appeal to the public for more money for the hospital, but with little success. One consultant, however, succeeded in securing a donation to sustain his service for a year, and another set up an appeal fund that has provided over £250 000 yearly in revenue to support the children's unit.

31

The crisis encouraged a deep analysis of strategy and structure. The most important question to be answered was whether clinicians should be concerned with the management of hospitals. The important characteristic of an NHS hospital is that it is cash limited, unlike a private hospital, in which income is related to activity. Clinicians need resources if they are to have clinical freedom. An authority that is cash limited will not transfer responsibility for management to a group that refuses to accept financial responsibility, nor will it readily accept or act on advice from a medical advisory committee if the members of the committee are not financially aware or accountable. After much debate the clinicians at Guy's Hospital reached an agreement with the district health authority whereby they would accept financial responsibility and accountability in return for management authority. Parenthetically, they also realised that if they could show that the hospital was efficient they would have a stronger voice in determining the allocation of resources at all levels in the NHS. There are, however, four principles that in our opinion govern the participation of clinicians in management.

Professional and management accountability are different

Unlike staff in most organisations, hospital staff are drawn from members of several very different professions. Nurses, administrators, scientists, engineers, catering staff, porters, accountants, personnel officers, clerical staff, and doctors all have their own professional organisations that determine training and set standards and to which they are accountable. Traditionally, hospitals have been administered by a trio of a doctor, a nurse, and an administrator, with help from other professional groups. The head of each professional group is concerned largely with the performance of his or her own department or function and has only a secondary concern for overall management, rather like a first violin player in an orchestra, with no director or conductor. General management has to be seen in the light of many different professional groups that comprise the staff of a hospital.[4] No one person can hope to understand, let alone lead, such an organisation. Mr Enoch Powell remarked recently that the Minister of Health has to accept advice from doctors without question whereas the Minister for Defence can contradict his generals.

Professional accountability must be protected, and certainly no interference by management in the care of a patient can or should be tolerated; the first responsibility of a doctor is to the patient. Management accountability is separate and different. The public has the right to know that the resources provided by taxation are being used efficiently and effectively and that everyone in the organisation is accountable managerially. In our structure staff continue to report professionally and are accountable to their seniors; thus all nurses are accountable to the director of nursing. Managerially, the final responsibility is held by the chairman of the board, who is a doctor, and the nurses, administrators, etc, are accountable finally to him; he in turn is accountable to the district general manager and the district health authority.

Responsibility and authority must be commensurate

Large hospitals are too complex to be managed centrally. We decentralised to 14 clinical directorates, each managed by a team of a nurse and a business manager and headed by a doctor. Each directorate manages its own affairs as far as possible and has its own doctors, nurses, clerical staff; scientists, technicians, records staff, etc. Each has its own ward or wards and organises its own admissions, outpatients, etc. Two thirds of our staff now report within these directorates. Budgets are set yearly, and there is a requirement to meet agreed targets of quantity and quality for patient care within the financial provision. Responsibility that is decentralised, however, must be accompanmied by the transfer of authority. If power without responsibility is dangerous then responsibility without authority is demoralising.

Lines of accountability should be as short as possible. The Salmon structure for nursing with its inbuilt "Chinese whispers" reduced the authority and managerial competence of ward sisters. In our structure clinical groups led by the ward sister and consultant have their own budgets and report to the clinical directorate concerned.

Part time commitment

Clinical practice requires practice, and clinicians in management should continue to maintain clinical duties for the benefit of their own professional futures and satisfaction and because they can bring their unique perspective to management only if they continue to be active clinically. Management and administration should not be confused. The clinician manager needs an administrator, who should be a colleague whose professional skills are valued. The relationship between the manager and the administrator can be viewed as similar to that between a minister and a permanent secretary.

Information and budgeting

Good management needs good information—for instance, I was taught that the first action to take when a patient with diabetic ketoacidosis was admitted was to telephone the staff of the clinical chemistry laboratory and enlist their support. Good management, however, also depends on doing the best you can with the information available. It is no use providing sophisticated information or clinical budgeting systems if there is no management structure that can use the information. Our policy has been to concentrate on getting the structure right. The new management board at Guy's Hospital, which started working in April 1985, inherited a yearly rate of overspending of about £5m. This was tackled by recognising that 60–70% of expenditure was on staff costs and that the key pieces of information that we lacked were how many people we employed and how much they earned. Overspending is best approached by reducing costs and then allowing activity to adjust rather than the reverse. Having identified the role of each employee, we then reduced staffing by about 10% over six months while doing our best to protect clinical activity. One of the key tasks of the NHS is to regain the post-1948 enthusiasm for treating as many patients as possible to an acceptable standard rather than being led by the need to balance the books. Balancing the books is essential but is not the purpose of the service. In the past three years we have reduced staffing by about 17% and expenditure by 15% (£7m yearly) but this year will treat nearly 40 000 in-patients—more than ever before.

Accountancy in the NHS is traditionally functionally based; thus nursing staff, medical staff, clerical staff, maintenance, and catering all have budgets even though they are mostly unmanageable by any one person. Reorganisation into multiprofessional management groups must be followed by management accountancy so that each of these groups is provided with accurate information concerning income and expenditure. The NHS should change from functional to management accountancy urgently. It takes time to set up these new systems, and the quality of the information improves only after an iterative process between the finance department and the manager. We hope that by April 1990 our clinical directorates and ward based clinical groups will receive monthly statements of expenditure set against budgets for staffing costs, other expenditure in the central sterile supply department, stores and supplies, drugs, repairs and maintenance, and consumables in pathology and radiology departments. The possibilities for improving efficiency should not be underestimated: a ward sister recently saved £5000 in nursing costs and £1300 in consumable costs on her ward in one month.

Quality

As long as patients cannot receive the treatment they need when they need it quantity must remain the most important aspect of quality in the NHS, but it should not be an excuse for poor quality. Improving quality can save money and improve clinical efficiency and effectiveness. Our decentralised outpatient appointment system, run by each firm's medical records officer and clinic clerk, has led to better spaced appointments with reduced waiting times, less crowding, and, therefore, less pressure on the staff, no missing notes, and no fewer patients. Preadmission clinics for surgery with regular reviews of waiting lists can lead to fewer operations being cancelled. High occupancy of beds does not necessarily mean higher patient throughput, and we all know hospitals where patients are admitted early simply to "protect the bed." These are all things where only the doctor "can reach the parts that other managers fail to reach." Medical audit or clinical review should also be encouraged as a means to improve clinical efficiency as well as effectiveness.[5]

Time

A common argument used against concerning clinicians with management is lack of time: it is worth asking, How much time is spent in committees? and Is this effort productive? Using your own and others' time efficiently is an essential quality of management. Much can be achieved by a telephone conversation, by being rigorous about reading and keeping only essential material, by not having lots of minutes, by stating when a meeting will end as well as when it will start, and by delegation. Again, however, it should be emphasised that time spent in determining operational policies is seldom wasted, and a well organised clinical service will release time and resources for caring for patients. Management time for clinicians can often be created outside clinical sessions: surgeons like to meet before breakfast whereas physicians seem to prefer to meet at dinner; lunchtime is a good time to meet the non-clinical staff.

Listening

As a manager it is easy to become desk bound and concerned with details to the extent that the main tasks pass you by. You should try to ensure that you keep definite periods free for visiting all parts of the hospital—"the best manure is the farmer's feet"— and you may find that visiting people in their own departments rather than meeting them in your office is useful and helps to put a problem into its proper context. You should be available to offer advice when problems occur is important, and in the long run this can save a lot of time for yourself and the whole organisation. Dealing with mail efficiently and promptly is important, and generally I try to ensure that my desk is clear at the end of each day.

Decisions and leadership

A good manager has to be decisive, but not all decisions will be correct for whatever reason, and there is often no harm in admitting that you were wrong and trying again. A good decision will command support among all those who have to implement it, and, indeed, they should have helped in formulating it. Often a properly led discussion will produce an obvious decision, at other times competing priorities will preclude a consensus, but the decision, once made, will still be carried through as long as everyone is satisfied that it has been properly reached.

A clinical manager has an important leadership role. Leadership implies that there are those who are prepared to follow. The clinical directors at Guy's and the chairman of the board are appointed not elected, but if it is clear that they have lost the support of their colleagues they have little option other than to resign and be replaced. Checks on the possible abuse of authority are important, and the British system of all consultants being created equal is too valuable to discard.

Incentives and motivation

The main defect of the NHS is the lack of incentive to good performance at all levels. Far too many people earn far too little and work far too ineffectively. We need the freedom to pay people according to performance and can look to do so by using the resources released by employing fewer people. Even under the present system a little imagination can be helpful, but changes in the all embracing and suffocating Whitley system are required urgently. A system is also required to make sure that efficient and effective hospitals and services are rewarded with more resources. Indeed, if under a cash limited system resources fail to benefit the patient then the NHS will inevitably stop being national. A good manager will be looking for ways to increase motivation and should not underestimate the devotion to patient care of all staff in the NHS. Most people who work in the service are proud of it and are underappreciated; showing that you, the manager, appreciate their efforts is vital.

Everyone in the organisation should understand their job, should know to whom they report, and should have their performance reviewed regularly to provide motivation, advice, and help. The flow of information up and down the organisation can be improved by a system of team briefing.[6] Social occasions are important, and an occasional chat over a drink can often be invaluable.

Nothing causes so much uncertainty or hostility in a hospital as a reorganisation of office, clinic, or ward space. None the less, it is vital that staff in management teams work near each other so that communication is facilitated. Key staff in the central management such as the clinician manager, chief administrator, director of nursing, financial director, and personnel director must have their offices near each other.

Training

I have already suggested that clinicians have more management experience than they might realise. They need to have a general appreciation of how the NHS works and the roles and skills of other professionals. Much can be learnt from informal discussions with finance staff, administrators, and personnel officers. Courses such as those run by the King's Fund College, the Royal College of Physicians, and the NHS Training Authority can be useful not only because of what is taught but also for the chance to meet others with similar responsibilities and to reflect on problems. They can also be useful in developing interpersonal skills and techniques for solving problems. Imagination is vital for solving problems but needs to be stimulated. Occasional sessions spent with colleagues in management, preferably in the evenings or off site so that interruptions are minimised, are useful to work out tactics and strategy and are usually educational. There is no body of knowledge, such as is required for a medical qualification, that has to be gained; thankfully, too, there are no exams worth taking, and we should restrict their creation.

Conclusion

This is a critical time for the NHS. There are powerful forces pressing for changes either to create more bureaucratic and political control or to move to a more market dominated system that is provided privately though subsidised publicly. Either way the service needs to be managed more competently. It is in the interests of patients as well as doctors that clinicians should participate in the management of their hospitals. A team approach that uses the skills of other professionals and shares the responsibility for management with other clinical colleagues by decentralisation offers the opportunity for clinicians to be managers without making it impossible for them to pursue clinical or academic practice. The NHS needs more money and a greater share of the national revenue. We are more likely to obtain this if we can show clinical efficiency and effectiveness and maintain the support of the public by providing a more personal and convenient service. Management is too important to be left to the others; doctors must play a part.

References

1 Drucker P F. *Management*. London: Pan Books, 1977.
2 Harvey-Jones J. *Making it happen*. London: Collins, 1988.
3 Peters T J, Wateman H. *In search of excellence: lessons from America's best run companies*. London: Harper and Row, 1982; 1: 360.

4 NHS Management Inquiry. *Report*. London: Department of Health and Social Security, 1983. (Griffiths report.)
5 Hoffenberg R. *Clinical freedom*. London: Nuffield Provincial Hospitals Trust, 1987; 1–105.
6 Grummitt J. *Team briefing*. 2nd ed. London: Industrial Society, 1988.

Choose a word processor

JOHN AINSLIE

Before you rush out and buy a word processor may I be so bold as to ask why you are parting with your money?

What word processing is—and isn't

The most obvious way to think of a word processor is as a rather clever typewriter that (*a*) allows you to enter all your text (letter, report, etc) on to a screen and edit it before you print it; (*b*) knows when to start new lines and new pages without you having to be bothered about such things; and (*c*) enables you to cover up all your typing errors without leaving your finished product an advertisement for Tipp-Ex. And when you've printed it out on your printer (while you type your next letter or drink a cup of tea) and it is still not to your liking you can go back and edit the original text and print it out again. And if your masterpiece of an article for the *BMJ* isn't appreciated by the folk at BMA House you can always retrieve it six months later, rewrite it, and try again. Word processors offer other bells and whistles as well, but my thumbnail sketch will do for now.

In deciding whether to invest in a word processing system of any kind there are two paramount questions. Firstly, do you do enough typing work to make it practical? No word processing is possible without some teach yourself sessions with the tutorial manual provided. Computers might be wonderful but they are not magic. If you can't remember how to do the basic operations from one work session to another then you do not have enough work to make a word processor worth while. Secondly, how much editing and re-editing do you do with the same script? If all you do is one off personal letters a word processor will show little advantage over an electric typewriter. Computers are best at doing repetitive tasks on the same data or on the same kind of data. The more your requirements fall into a standard pattern on standard paper the easier it will be to get the dumb machine to do it right each time. Word processors will do more complicated tasks like tables, columns, and personalised standard letters, even elementary arithmetic, but such things are not for the novice user. Some tasks are actually easier on typewriters—typing on envelopes, for example.

Hard and soft word processors

Up to 1980 there was only one kind of word processor, made by Wordplex, AES, and some others. This was a machine designed for one function—word processing—and essentially for one market—the busy secretarial office.

Their successors for the less intensive user are, on the one hand, sophisticated typewriters with one line screens along which your script dances (and can be corrected) before being printed out and, on the other hand, full screen and typewriter outfits with diskettes to keep your text on for later retrieval. The first system will save on your Tipp-Ex but will not save your text; the second may well be cumbersome—and make sure you can read the screen easily. Olivetti and Brother have a whole range of machines from one extreme to the other. What they have in common is that they are essentially single purpose: word processing or bust. Note too, that diskettes from a hard wired word processor of this kind cannot be read by microcomputers or by machines of a different make.

The true microcomputer has a more flexible approach but comes out more expensive in the long run when you add all its bits together. As delivered it cannot do anything useful at all, but you can install software (that is, off the shelf programs on diskettes) for it to run: accounting, budgeting, record keeping, and, of course, word processing, all capable of being installed separately as and when the computer owner wants. This software is easier to produce and develop than the hard wired word processing facility offered on dedicated machines, and different vendors can offer rival products to run on the same machine.

Of course someone had to come up with a standard machine specification on which to run all this software. "Big Blue," alias IBM, produced its personal computer (PC) in 1981, and most software has claimed to be "PC compatible" ever since. Only Apple with its Macintosh series has sustained a competitive challenge, but at a higher price—and at the price of incompatibility. Atari and

BBC were conceived for educational rather than business use. Like it or not, "PC compatible" software has the lion's share of the business word processing market.

Caveat emptor

If all you want is a clever typewriter you shouldn't have any difficulty in installing it, but the more clever it is the more time you will need to discover how to unlock its secrets.

When it comes to computer systems, however, I would urge you most strongly to seek a dealer who will set up your entire system (hardware and software) in the shop, test it, and demonstrate it to you to your satisfaction before you accept delivery. The word processing software (or any other software) will almost certainly have been supplied by a third party, not the makers of the computer, and the printer for your system will probably hail from somewhere else, so it is most important that the whole lot be assembled and "configured" so that the word processing software communicates properly with the computer and the printer. Check that when you press the £ sign key on the keyboard a £ sign duly appears on the screen and also on the printed copy (most computers are designed in the United States, most printers in Japan . . .). Will you want to use accented characters for foreign languages, or fractions, or to create borders round your text? Most word processing software will allow you to do these things, but they have to be set up in advance in their own peculiar way.

Once you are satisfied with what your dealer is offering you can get it delivered and set it up in your own home, office, or wherever you want to use it. And—this is the vital bit—reach a clear understanding about what happens when things go wrong. Will the dealer come to you? Within how many hours of your call? How long will it be before you are up and running again? If the dealer doesn't undertake this support personally, a maintenance contract with a third party may be offered, in which case it behoves you to find out something about the maintenance and where your dealer's support ends and the maintainer's starts.

Incidentally, you are much less likely to get this kind of dealer and maintenance support if you buy a machine at the bargain end of the market, like an Amstrad—the dealer's margins are just too small to make it worth his while. But ask your dealer about the Opus range.

Choosing a computer system

The computer comprises three units: screen, keyboard, and system unit. All system units have at least one diskette (or floppy disc) drive for loading the machine and backing up the data. You need at least a two drive system: the second drive may be for another diskette, but I would recommend a hard disc machine, which will contain your entire filing cabinet permanently, removing the worry of having to find the right diskette with the bit of information you want. A hard disc machine can be started up by simply switching on, whereas a two diskette unit always needs some fiddling with diskettes to get it started and to do any work on it. When you are using the word processing software the size, spacing, and quality of the typeface displayed on the screen are important, as is the feel of the keyboard (make sure all the keys work at the same finger pressure).

The printer—The cheapest printers are dot matrix ones; when these are used in "near letter quality" mode they produce a reasonable quality of print, adequate for letters but not up to the quality of a carbon ribbon electric typewriter. Daisywheel printers produce excellent quality type but are slower and noisier. Laser printers are likely to be outside the personal budget. There are some quiet, reasonably priced and high quality printers that use ink jet or other new technology, but find out how expensive the refills are for them.

The word processing software—For this, as for everything else, cost is related to quality. There may be some cheap word processing software that comes free with the computer but it may well be limited in scope. Of the best known word processing software, WordStar was in danger of being left behind, but the 2000 version and release 5 are endeavouring to keep it up to its rivals, notably Microsoft's Word and WordPerfect. These last two are top of the market products costing about £400 each; WordPerfect is the market leader and, incidentally, the standard software used at BMA House. Incidentally, be wary of brand new versions of any software: these are prone to development bugs. It is better to opt for established "bedded down" versions of programs which you can update later if necessary.

You and your data

You now have your word processor or micro ready on your desk and are about to entrust your finest thoughts to its tender mercies. The hard disc in the machine (or your collection of diskettes) is about to become your filing cabinet: it is imperative that you know how to take security copies from it, otherwise you may one day find it locked up for good or totally rubbished. If your filing cabinet is important enough for you to entrust its contents to a computer, taking care of it is even more important. That applies even when you are in the middle of your editing; you should back up to disc or diskette frequently so that when your dog trips over the power cable you will lose only a page or two and not your whole morning's work.

You also need to secure the data in your machine against unauthorised access. Most computers are equipped with a key-operated locking mechanism which prevents the machine being started when locked. Alternatively, IBM offers a password entry protection facility. Of course, your original software and backup diskettes should be locked away; particularly sensitive data files can be made "invisible" or encrypted by use of suitable software, though you have to decrypt them each time you wish to work on them.

Incidentally, personal information, including names and addresses, may be covered by the Data Protection Act 1986. This means that any person may require you to provide details of all the data you may have about him or her on your computer.

Over to you

There are other goodies on offer like spelling checkers (which make hilarious nonsense of proper names) and thesauruses (also useful for solving crosswords). You can even get software to comment on your writing style, but that might be too much for the blood pressure. Unfortunately, you still have to write the text yourself.

File reprints

MICHAEL MARMOT

Like most academics, I will shamelessly forget our ignorance and presume actually to lecture as if I knew something, but I have no such pretensions about filing references. I could hardly be counted an expert. I have not a single slide on the topic.

Why me? It cannot be because the editor secretly visited my office and was impressed by the reference files. Why not ask an information technologist? If the editor wanted to know how to prepare breakfast, surely he would be better advised to approach Anton Mossiman than to ask me. I *do* know how to prepare breakfast in a way that suits me. But I would never be so arrogant as to suggest that it is *the* way to prepare breakfast.

A system that works for me is the approach I shall take in describing how to file references: not the Anton Mossiman approach to the supreme breakfast, but the approach of a humble breakfast eater who sometimes misses a breakfast, or finds that he has run out of oranges when his need is great. It is an occupational hazard of epidemiologists to be concerned with warnings of risks. Nevertheless, in this area, at least, I am much more comfortable with a list of don'ts than a list of do's. As everyone knows, to sculpt an elephant from a block of marble, you chip away all the bits that don't look like a bit of the elephant and what you are left with is an elephant. If you get rid of some of the bad practices what you might be left with is a system that works for you. In case that is not enough I shall even describe two systems I have used: one off and one on the computer.

Why file references?

There are perhaps three main reasons why people accumulate reprints: photocopying takes less time than reading; the contents can be referred to at a later date; and a photocopy makes it easier to cite a reference when writing a paper.

The first is ignoble, and wasteful of both time and resources. Don't photocopy an article because you think it might be interesting and you haven't the time to read it now. There may be one or two people left working in health or higher education who still have access to all the secretarial or clerical help they feel they need, but they are not among my acquaintances. It is not a good use of your or a secretary's time to photocopy an article on the off-chance that you might have the time to read it later. Read it now, and then if you feel you must have it, obtain a copy.

It may be that the reprint-type services work well for some people—that is, those where you survey the contents pages of all known journals and fire off a shower of reprint requests every week. They don't work well for me. As with photocopying, it is easier to fire off a reprint request than to read an article. How many, I wonder, of the reprints dispatched in response to the requests that come thudding through the letter box actually get read?

But you are not that sort of person I hear you say. You do read first and then accumulate, but do you overdo it? It is very tempting to keep everything that may be of future interest, or that could be used in future teaching, research, or practice. But that is very expensive of time and storage space. Might it not be better to go back to the library occasionally than to accumulate vast quantities of references that are never again to be seen. Be selective. I know to my cost. When I decided to put my references on computer (more of that anon), it was so expensive (time) that I only entered about a third of them. In the subsequent six months I have had little need to access the dormant two thirds.

Why do you need a system?

Let us take what is, for me, a typical writing experience. You are writing a paper on alcohol and blood pressure. You need to remind yourself of how your results fit in with those of published papers. You pull out all the papers you have on the subject and you place your results in an appropriate context. Then comes the fun part. You prepare the text and tables and bask in a warm glow of achievement. The paper is finished, and you can now move on to preparing a lecture on depression and cancer. But it is not finished. There is the job of the references. You copy them off the papers you have, struggling with the spelling of foreign names and the opaque intricacies of the Vancouver system. As any editor will report, you do this appallingly badly. If you applied the same standard of accuracy to your data as you do to your references, your paper would, rightly, be bounced. In fact, it is possible that the reviewer of your manuscript may assume that you do apply the same sloppy standards to your data and bounce it anyway.

But then there are the references you don't have. You remember reading a paper by Mendeleev on vodka and blood pressure and you can neither find the paper nor remember the journal, nor for that matter whether it was by Mendeleev *et al*, or by *et al* and Mendeleev, or was it Stanislavsky? The infuriating thing is that you know that this very paper has been in your hands as you sat at this very desk and you can even picture the graphs of blood pressure showing a J-shaped relation with alcohol consumption. It then dawns on you that you pulled this paper out when you needed Mendeleev's address for a list you were compiling of European investigators interested in cooperative work, and if only you can remember where that folder is. . . . There are also, of course, the three papers you lent to, to . . . to . . . ?

Even that hurdle is overcome. You send off the paper and now the work is finished. Regrettably, it is not. You are already deep into all the things you put off while you were finishing the paper, including the lecture on depression and cancer (which looks now like being a short lecture: it is depressing), and have not the time for anything as menial as refiling the reprints. That way madness lies. Next time you want to find those reprints, and experience shows that you tend to cite those same papers repeatedly, where will they be?

Entropy increases

The message of this story can be summarised by remembering the second law of thermodynamics: the universe tends to entropy. And this is nowhere more evident than with references. More specifically, remember a few don'ts:

- don't delay in refiling reprints;
- don't let reprints out for more than the time it takes a colleague to read them—they will drift;

- don't construct a reference in Vancouver style more times than
  you need;
- don't delay any longer in setting up a proper system.

We have one research fellow in the department with an IQ of
4000 who has read everything, forgotten nothing, and has copies
strewn all over the floor, mingled with used squash gear, piles of
computer printout, and goodness knows what. Most people going
into his room can scarcely find the door, but in a race to find a reprint he always wins. Even he is now setting up a system that
ordinary mortals would recognise as such. It is essential.

What type of system?

This can be split into two (1) the system of filing the reprints;
and (2) the filing of the references to them. The two are related.

By topic

The simplest system of filing reprints is to cluster them by topic.
All your references to do with alcohol and blood pressure go into a
file or box on that subject. This works (i) if you have not too many
reprints, or (ii) an infallible mmeory. The drawbacks of this simple
system are obvious. When you come to prepare a paper on the
public health response to the problems of alcohol, you have to
search through the blood pressure file, the coronary heart disease
file, the cancer file, mental illness, economics, motor vehicle accidents, plus the separate file you have on *BMJ* articles by Smith.
Will you really remember which file yielded up which article, so
that you can replace them in the appropriate one? This method
might be appropriate for a topic that you might start to be interested in but you are not yet sure. For example, you throw everything you have read on the destruction of medical education by
underfunding into one box, pending serious review one day
(perhaps after you have been made redundant).

In alphabetical order

Most of us find the pressure to have a more systematic way
somewhat irresistible. My choice was to file all reprints in alphabetical order by the first author's name. Others assign each reprint
a number as it comes in and file them in numerical order. Both
systems should be supplemented by either a card or computer

system of keeping references. The advantage, I find, of the alphabetical system of filing is that you can bypass your card system if need be and go straight to your files to find the paper by Mendeleev (provided he really was the first author), without first having to look up the paper's accession number.

References

My old system was cards. Two cards for each reprint: one filed by alphabetical order of first author, the other by topic. Yet, what if something belonged in two or more topics? I just had to remember. But at least I had two chances: either remember the author's name or the topic under which I had catalogued the card.

Computers

I was a reluctant convert to modern technology. I have a very elegant pencil and a yen for beautiful white paper, but in the end I shelled out a different type of Yen for an electronic friend. One of the reasons was that I could no longer bear the pain of the references at the end of papers. The finding, the typing, the proof reading (how do you spell Mendeleef?), or the changing from Vancouver style to some other form for that book chapter.

There are, no doubt, several reference systems and you will have to look elsewhere for a thorough review.[1] The one we purchased, Reference Manager (Research Information Systems, 1991 Village Park Way, Encenitas, California 9204, USA) works well, and scores quite highly in the *Which?* type comparisons.[1] You enter your references once on the Reference Manager system and **never** have to type that reference again. You can set the system up to produce your references in various styles, and when you enter the reference you also enter several key words. When searching for a reference, you can search on any of the authors, not only the first (you really can look for *et al* and Mendeleev), but on journal, key words, and title, or accession number.

The part that you really like to bore your friends with comes when writing the paper. In your unique database, *et al* and Mendeleev has the number 4006 because it was the 4006th reference that you entered in your Reference Manager file. In the text of your paper you cite the reference as {4006}. When you have finished the final final draft of your paper for the *BMJ*, the Reference Manager goes through the paper and replaces all the {4006}s.[2] It then constructs the reference list for you in *BMJ* format. Miraculous.

When I started using this, regrettably it cut my productivity by half. But that is my experience of each faltering step I have taken with the computer. When you get over the inevitable teething troubles that are almost always because you have done something stupid, the thing really works. I do now have my key references on the hard disc of my Toshiba Laptop and can actually keep editing anywhere. It keeps your mind off which part of the Boeing was last reported to have fallen off.

The other big advantage of a system like the Reference Manager is that you can lend references without parting with the reprints and having to worry about entropy. Anyone in the department can access my database to look up references and vice versa.

In the end that has to be the recommendation of this flawed, imperfect breakfast eater. One final word of warning. When you do decide to switch over to a computerised system, don't get caught halfway. The most frustrating position to be in is with a substantial slice of your references on the computer, but never the ones you want.

I had hoped to get to the end of this without any expertise at all, only bitter experience. In the end, my insecurity got the better of me and I sought the reassurance of an expert. John Eyers, assistant librarian at the London School of Hygiene and Tropical Medicine, agrees with the choice of Reference Manager, but warns that the system needs to be managed. If more than one person is inputting references someone has to make sure that they are correctly input and a standard set of key words is used. He also supplied a useful reference.[2] But now is the time to set up your own limited, database.

References

1   Wachtel R E. Personal bibliographic databases. *Science* 1987; **235**: 1093–6.
2   Heeks R. *Personal bibliographic indexes and their computerisation.* London: Taylor Graham, 1986.

Write the annual report of the director of public health

JOHN MIDDLETON, KATHY BINYSH, VALERIE
CHISHTY, GEORGE POLLOCK

Introduction

The Acheson Report on *Public Health in England* defines public
health as, "the art and science of the prevention of disease, the pro-
longation of life and the promotion of health through the organised
efforts of society".[1] The recent health circular, HC (88) 64, requires health authorities to appoint a director of public health
(DPH) and for this director to produce an annual report on the
state of the public health in the district or region.[2]

Before the health service was reorganised in 1974, local authority medical officers of health had a statutory obligation to produce
annual health reports. In these the health profile of the local population was discussed, the factors influencing this analysed, and
recommendations made for action to prevent and treat disease and
promote health. In practice, many of these reports had become
indigestible catalogues of mortality and notifiable infections, and
after 1974 they stopped being produced to a large extent.

The reintroduction of the annual health report was one of many
unimplemented recommendations of the Black report.[3] In the
1980s there has been a resurgence of interest in health profiles for
districts from the local level. These "local Black reports" have
shown how adverse social conditions cause ill health and per-
petuate inequalities. Such reports have come from community
medicine departments in health authorities,[4-10] from local
authorities,[11-13] and from pressure groups, trade unions, and political organisations.[14-15] Some of these have been heavily influenced

by the World Health Organisation European targets for Health For All.[16]

The reintroduction of annual health reports will not, in itself, improve public health. The reports must be used as a basis for organised efforts to promote health at district and regional level. The reports must also become a focus within the health service planning cycle to enable the available health service resources to be appropriately targeted to meet needs effectively. Explicit in HC (88) 64 is the expectation that directors of public health will take part in the development of indicators of outcome of health care procedures.

This article draws on our experience in preparing and using our report *The Health of Coventry*.[4] It also draws on the proceedings of the December 1988 conference at the London School of Hygiene and Tropical Medicine, *The annual report on the public health: from idea to reality* (unpublished).

Aims and objectives

The DPH will need to determine the important issues for the district or region and thence broad aims for each year's report. The broad aims might include those cited in the figure.

The DPH will devise specific objectives from these broad aims. The aims of the report may include elements of all of the above: the emphasis will reflect the different local needs.

The aims of the report will determine for whom (besides the health authority) it is written and how it is written. It will also determine the size of the intended distribution and this will in turn influence whether the eventual report is photocopied or printed. The audience will include lay people and professionals; the written style will therefore need to be uncomplicated while the data used will need to be as precise as possible. The style should be non-sexist and sensitive to local cultural and ethnic minority needs. It may be necessary to include at least a summary and recommendations translated into appropriate languages.

The first annual report may differ from subsequent editions in that the DPH may wish to adopt a broad brush approach and comment on the full range of locally available health information. Addressing three or four main themes, however, can be a more effective means of concentrating attention on those areas the DPH feels should be the priorities.

Possible aims for the annual health report

- 1 To act as the stimulus or focus for multiagency work to promote public health.
- 2 To draw attention to social problems affecting health which can only be resolved by action by other local agencies, or by national action.
- 3 To draw attention to particular health service deficiencies to influence planning and resource allocation within the health authority.
- 4 To "market public health" to show the work done by the department of public health medicine, indicating its relevance to decisions being taken by the health authority and other agencies, and advertising its expertise as a resource for the local community.
- 5 To report local health studies undertaken during the year and recommend action based on these studies.
- 6 To report local epidemiological artefacts and advise on further research needed.
- 7 To report and restate public health successes such as fluoridation of water supplies or Clean Air Acts.
- 8 To act as an archive for reference in the future.

In each section of the *Health of Coventry* we included a précis of the evidence on health implications of housing, employment, and unemployment, and so on. This widened the lay interest in the report and had the unforeseen effect of increasing the understanding of public health of some senior health service managers.

Content of the report

If annual reports are to be of any value local "sovereignty" must be protected. Prescribed minimum data sets or department of health or regional DPH directives on content will immediately destroy the main function of these reports, which is to assess local needs and make recommendations for local action. Should the Department of Health require standardised information for its own purposes, it has the information technology and supply from which to do this. Measures of outcomes can be developed and presented in a similar format to that used for performance indicator packages; these data could then be used by districts and regions, if appropriate, in their annual reports.

In the *Health of Coventry* we progressed from demography, through major social influences of health, to routine health service data—that is, our order of importance (table 1).[4] The content is likely to be predominantly from routine sources of data; some of these are suggested in table 1. One off local studies can be included or quoted in the report. As the annual report becomes more established, we would expect such local studies to assume a prominent role and further enhance the local relevance of the report. Health service performance indicators are likely to be relevant in the annual report only where they indicate unmet needs and unnecessary suffering in the community.

Computer mapping programmes are becoming more widely available at district and regional level and offer great potential for presenting local health information by electoral ward or enumeration district.[17] Any data that can be postcoded can be presented in these graphics packages. Care is needed in presenting and interpreting data such as standardised mortality ratios by ward as the numbers involved will often be very small. These data should at least be aggregated over three or five years. The figures should also be accompanied by confidence intervals; alternatively, only the outlying wards can be shown.

TABLE 1—*Possible title headings for an annual health report, subject areas, and possible sources of information for local use*

1 *Demography:*
Population: at census; estimates; predictions; crude birth rate; crude mortality; fertility; single parent families; migration; ethnic minorities. [Office of Population Censuses and Surveys (OPCS) Census, Local Authority Planning and Information, Regional Health Authority Statistics Department (RHA)]

2 *Major determinants of health:*
Housing: housing "spaces", private, council, other; overcrowding, lacking basic amenities (census). Housing condition surveys; council waiting lists; homelessness; medical priority for rehousing [local authority (LA), homelessness agencies] *Poverty:* benefit claimants [Department of Social Security (DSS)] housing benefit claimants [indicator of very low income–LA]; percentage of unskilled workers (census); local poverty action groups and Low Pay Unit surveys; *Employment:* census of employment by standard industrial groupings (Department of Employment, LA Economic Units or Planning and Information); employment by socioeconomic groups (Census); industrial accidents [Health and Safety Executive, Hospital Activity Analysis (HAA)]. *Unemployment:* (LA Economic Units, DSS); water supply, quality and sanitation (Water Authority Reports, LA technical services/city engineers) *Education:* provision of nursery education; school population; percentage of school leavers entering higher education (LA education department) *Violence/personal security:* crime statistics (county councils or Metropolitan Police Authorities)

TABLE I—*continued*

3 *Hazards:*
Fires (county councils or metropolitan fire and civil defence authorities) *Pollution:* air monitoring and hazardous materials surveys [LA Environmental Health Departments (EHD)] water quality and pollution incidents (LA and water authorities). Food hygiene (LA EHD). *Environmental control:* pests, public health nuisances (LA EHD)

4 *Maternal and child health:*
Obstetric care; birthweight; congenital abnormalities; perinatal and infant deaths; legal abortions; [District health authority (DHA) and RHA information departments]; OPCS, notifiable infectious disease (LA, DHA) and immunisations; child abuse [LA social services (SSD)]; home and road accident statistics (additional data from LA EHD and police authorities) dental health (DHA local surveys of missing, decayed, and filled teeth in the school populations)

5 *Physical and mental handicap:*
Physical disablement, blindness and deafness registers (LA-SSD). Local surveys and proxy measures from national studies

6 *Adult health:*
Indicators from primary care (Royal College of General Practitioners spotter practices, local practice databases and reports) contraceptive use (DHA); prescriptions for major groupings of pharmaceuticals [Prescriptions Pricing Authority (PPA)] notifiable infectious disease; accidents; AIDS; sexually transmitted diseases; local information from lifestyle surveys, coronary heart disease risk factors. Smoking related diseases and coronary heart diseases (information similar to that presented for districts in the Health Education Authority reports "The Big Kill" and "Broken Hearts") home, road and work accidents statistics; drugs (Local drug agencies, LA-SSD Home Office statistics, Accident department and HAA, PPA, and Family Practitioner Committees). *Alcohol:* (local agencies and social services, HAA, extrapolate national estimates for local proxy measures)

7 *Major uses of hospital specialties:*
Major causes of hospital admission; major uses of hospital facilities; hospital performance; mental health. Standardised hospitalisation rates can be calculated by ward (DHA, RHA, DOH and John Yates Performance Indicator packages, HAA, Hospital Inpatient Enquiry, Mental Health Inquiry)

8 *Major causes of death:*
Mortality statistics, numbers (OPCS–SD25/VS1 series) rates over time, standardised mortality ratios by ward for major conditions, 3 or 5 year aggregated data, for all ages and for selected ages. 15–64, with confidence intervals (can be supplied by regional statistics departments but requires checking)

9 *Special reports/local research*

10 *Summary of findings and consequent recommendations**

11 *References/sources*

12 *Acknowledgements*

* In the case of Coventry, two chapters on health promotion priorities and Health For All in Coventry by the year 2000.

One off local studies, reports required by the AIDS Control Act 1987, hospital performance reports and reports of the Public Health Department's own activities could be included as "special reports" or appendices. There may be special subjects of peculiar relevance to a district, such as the foundry industry in Sandwell.[17]

The report must make recommendations to be adopted and "owned" by the agencies to which it is addressed. The report cannot be solely for reference purposes or for the archive.

Production of the report

The *Health of Coventry* was written in three months: typesetting, proof reading, and printing took a further three months.

A minimum of six months is required to produce an annual report. For the single handed DPH this may sound like an inordinate amount of time, particularly with other competing calls on his or her time. The preparation of the drafts of the report may be the shortest stage, however, while the longest time may be spent when copy is at the printers. Much of the work of assembling data should be delegated to the district or regional information department. Non-public health doctors can be recruited to write sections of the report.

At the outset, it is advisable to draw up a schedule for the production of the report. Research tasks and sections to be written should be assigned. It is advisable to write to non-NHS agencies for the data required as a first step; while awaiting that information, NHS data can be assembled, processed, and interpreted,

---

Panel: *Suggested timetable for the production of the annual health report*

April: Planning meeting: agree main priority areas; assign tasks of data collection, processing, and writing; agree special reports/local research for inclusion; agree programme of production

Write for information required from non-NHS sources

Undertake literature searches on main themes

Assess available NHS data and prepare first drafts text

May: Major period of report writing

Collate information and correspondence from outside agencies

June: DPH convenes editorial meeting: review of first draft; formulation of conclusions/recommendations; agree "target" organisations and individuals for eventual distribution; start to formulate plan for steering report launch in the most constructive manner

Advance notices for member seminars; preparations for other seminars; (if you wish councillors to attend, arrangements are required with the local authority director of finance to ensure councillor's expenses are payable)

"Medical editor" assumes control of project, editing content and providing consistent style

IF PRODUCING IN BOOKLET FORM FINAL DRAFT TO GO TO GRAPHICS ARTIST/ TYPESETTING FIRST WEEK IN JULY

July: Annual AIDS reports required: submit to regional health authority but also include in the annual report

OPCS mortality statistics from previous year expected: can just about be incorporated, but with little time for processing and interpretation

Arrange summary/conclusions in translation for ethnic minorities

DON'T USE A GRAPHIC ARTIST WHO CANNOT ARRANGE TRANSLATIONS

In parallel, prepare short popular version or leaflet

Start to prepare visual aids for presentations/allow eight weeks for poster paper

August: Produce final word processed/desk-top publishing draft

Send to printers

Proof read typeset version twice

Printers

Prepare distribution address labels

Prepare press release

September: Final arrangements for member seminars; calling notices

Arrangements for public seminars and press conference

October: Publication

Presentation to health authority

formatted for graphs and tables and the accompanying script prepared.

All the text should be put on a word processor for easy editing. A "medical editor", usually the DPH, is required to supervise the content, ensure a consistent literary style and consistent statements and figures throughout the text. Someone else should proof read. If possible, that person can also act as "administrative editor" to supervise the layout, printing, and distribution.

The choice of presentation and style and the printing resources available to the DPH will determine the time taken before the report is finally produced. *The Health of Coventry* was phototypeset and all the graphs were redrawn by a graphic artist. Desktop publishing software packages are now widely available for around £200 and would obviate the need for and the cost of professional typesetting. Desk-top publishing needs to be used with a laser printer, however (cost around £2000), and by an experienced operator for high quality results.

If large quantities of the report are to be produced the marginal cost of printing becomes smaller and may be less than photocopying. Printing also allows a much more polished and professional finish to be achieved. Annual health reports should be professionally finished and sufficiently glossy to read, without being ostentatious.

The central Birmingham health report cost £2650 for 1000 copies in 1987 (Evans M, personal communication). *The Health of Coventry* cost £5500 in 1985 for 2000 copies. Both have "broken even" through sales to other interested health authorities, some agencies within districts, and to private sources. The opportunities for sales within the health service will decline as these reports become more commonplace. *The Health of Coventry* would probably cost about £10 000 to produce in 1989, but this would still only be an actual cost of £5 per copy (and half the cost of photocopying the original draft).

Publication of the report

The annual health report must be presented to the health authority in full public session. The launch should be a media event. A press release should be prepared while the report is at the printers. Distribution lists can also be drawn up at this time (table II). A decision is needed about how many complementary copies are to be distributed and who is to be charged.

The report is intended to be the DPH's independent professional advice to the health authority, but it would clearly be an empty report if it were to be presented outside the context of the

TABLE II—*Possible distribution for the annual health report*

Health authority members
Senior officers, heads of department, health authority
One copy per ward, department, health centre and clinic
Medical executive committee members
District medical committee members
Nursing professional advisory committee members
Staff trade union representatives
Medical and nursing education centre libraries
Hospital patient libraries
Reception areas (fixed copies)

Family practitioner committee members
One copy per GP practice
Local medical committee members
Local dentists, pharmacists, and opticians committee members

Community health council members
Joint consultative committee members

Members of parliament
Representatives of all political parties
All councillors
All local authority chief officers
Additional copies to other key local authority officers, particularly those who have
    provided information such as planning, economic, and information departments,
    road safety, environmental health, social services registers. All school
    headteachers and one copy for school libraries
Social services and housing district/neighbourhood offices
One copy for each general library

Police, fire, and ambulance chiefs
Coroners

Community relations council members
Voluntary services coordinator (and to all agencies on mailing list if available)
Church organisations

Chamber of Commerce members
Other industrial or business organisations
Manpower services commission
Enterprise agencies and development corporations
Trades council members

Regional health authority: director of public health, general manager, chairman

Department of Health: chief medical officer, health minister
British Library (if published in book form)

planning process and without the support and commitment of general managers and other senior officers of the health authority. DPHs will therefore need to determine their most appropriate course of action to secure managers' cooperation when publishing their annual reports.

It is likely that October will become the most appropriate time for publication of the annual report, to coincide with the formulation of the operational plans and budget setting for the following year. This timing might allow for the incorporation of the OPCS mortality statistics for the previous year which are generally published in July. This would put the report on a very tight time schedule. We believe the annual report should contain the most recent available data to enable it to be published to influence planning decisions in health authorities. Most causes of death are not changing sufficiently rapidly to affect planning for a maximum of three years ahead. The health report should be for the year in which it is published and not the year from which the data are drawn.

Major public health reports could be produced to influence the health authority strategic plans (every 10 years) and in the year of the mid-strategy review.

Uses of the report

Ashton has described the use of his report on health in Mersey as the starting point for community based health promotion initiatives.[18] Table III shows some of the uses to which we put the *Health of Coventry*: these have been described elsewhere.[19]

The scale of activity generated by the first report is clearly greater than that likely to result from subsequent reports, but public health physicians must capitalise on the interest that is likely to be generated on the publication of their first "new public health" reports, and be prepared to take on the additional work with vigour and enthusiasm. Subsequent reports need to be sufficiently different to sustain the interest of writer and reader and sufficiently consistent to enable sustained public health initiatives to develop.

Conclusions

Ashton has described the health report as the "community diagnosis"[18]; as with the clinical diagnosis, it is not an end in itself—it provides the information on which to base the "community treatment". It is not sufficient to produce glossy reports on the problems faced by our communities; it is necessary to use the information in these reports to campaign on behalf of the public

TABLE III—*Possible uses for the annual health report*[18, 19]

Presentations:
Health authority
Family practitioner committee
Community health council   formal public presentation
Joint consultative committee   and members seminars
Full council and relevant
   council committees

District management board, health authority
Chief officers meeting, local authority

Medical advisory committee meetings
Nursing professional advisory committee meetings
Other professional and technical committee meetings
Staff trade union committee meetings

Additional seminars offered for all health service staff
Formal postgraduate medical education presentations
Schools of nursing and midwifery

General offer of presentations for schools, political, church, trade union, industrial,
   commercial, voluntary, community and ethnic minority organisations (to be
   circulated with report copies or flyer)

Press conference(s)
Formal district or regionwide seminar to publicise findings and explore
   recommendations[20]
Videos
Follow up seminars on specific issues[21]
Popular, short version of the report, for separate publication, or as feature in local
   authority or health authority free paper

Service planning, health services, local authority and other agencies:
Incorporation of major recommendations into operational or strategic plans for
   health authorities

Consideration of major recommendations in planning by family practitioner
   committees, local authorities, and other agencies

Development of outcome measures as part of the information strategy/consumer
   affairs/quality of service strategy[22]

Development of joint activities through the joint consultative committee, a joint
   health promotion group, or through advice to local authority health
   committee[12, 18–20]

Advertise services of department as a resource for information for community
   based health promotion campaigns

---

health and to involve people in their own local initiatives to improve health. The development of the annual report on the state of the public health provides the information on which broad based health promotion can be established.

References

1 Department of Health. *Public health in England (the Acheson report).* London: HMSO, 1988.
2 Department of Health. *Health of the population: responsibilities of health authorities.* Health circular, HC (88) 64. London: DHSS, 1988.
3 Townsend P, Davidson N, eds. *Inequalities in health: the Black report.* Harmondsworth: Penguin, 1982.
4 Binysh K, Chishty V, Middleton J, Pollock G. *The health of Coventry.* Coventry: Coventry health authority, 1985.
5 Bloomsbury Department of Community Medicine. *Health for all.* Bloomsbury: Bloomsbury health authority, 1985.
6 Ashtomn J. *Health in Mersey: a review.* Liverpool: University of Liverpool, 1984.
7 Central Birmingham Department of Community Medicine. *A picture of health.* Birmingham: Central Birmingham health authority, 1987.
8 Lewisham and North Southwark Department of Community Medicine. *Dying before our time: health in Lewisham and North Southwark health authority.* London: London and Southwark health authority, 1987.
9 Boulton G, Roberts R E. *Mid Glamorgan: deprivation and health.*Cardiff: Mid-Glamorgan health authority, 1985.
10 Community Physicians of the Manchester Joint Consultative Committee. *Health inequalities in Manchester.* Manchester: Manchester joint consultative committee, 1982.
11 Thunhurst C. *Poverty and health in the city of Sheffield.* Sheffield: Sheffield city council environmental health department, 1984.
12 Fryer P. A healthy city strategy three years on—the case of Oxford city council. *Health Promotion* 1988; **3**: 213–17.
13 Nottingham City Council Health Unit. *Health for all in Nottingham.* Nottingham: Nottingham city council, 1988.
14 West of Scotland Politics of Health Group. *Glasgow: health of a city.* Glasgow: West of Scotland politics of health group, 1984.
15 Gardner K, Mumby S, eds. *Liverpool's state of health.* Liverpool: Merseyside communist party, 1984.
16 WHO EURO. *Targets in support of European health for all by the year 2000.* Copenhagen: European office of the world health organisation, 1985.
17 Sandwell Department of Public Health. *Life and death in Sandwell.* West Bromwich: Sandwell health authority, 1989.
18 Ashton J. Health in Mersey—an exercise in community diagnosis. *Health Education J* 1985; **44**: 178–80.
19 Binysh K, Chisty V, Middleton J, Pollock G. The health of Coventry—use of a health profile to stimulate community health promotion. *Health Education J* 1989 (in press)
20 Binysh K, Chisty V, Middleton J, Pollock G. *Coventry health 2000: proceedings of a conference on health for Coventry by the year 2000.* Coventry: Coventry health authority, 1986.

21 Coventry safe driving team. Coventry: a no drinking driving city by the year 2000? *Br Med J* 1987; **295**: 71–2.
22 Middleton J. A discussion paper on outcomes for a non-teaching district. *Community Medicine* 1987; **9**: 343–9.

Please an editor

ALISTAIR BREWIS

Editors are easily pleased—but not often. All they require is a manuscript which describes work which is sound, original, interesting and preferably controversial, and which is presented to their journal before any other. Matters of presentation are a secondary consideration for authors who are able to provide articles which meet these criteria because editors are prepared to take a great deal of trouble improving the arrangement of really excellent work. Most articles submitted to journals are, however, no more than reasonably sound, fairly original, and moderately interesting, and in these circumstances the editor's pleasure will be similarly moderate. The chances of acceptance are then influenced by whether or not the article incurs the editor's displeasure. There are very many ways of doing this.

Preparing for the selected journal

Authors like to have their work published in what are regarded as worthy journals, and there is an unofficial pecking order in most specialties and even among general journals. Even though editors know perfectly well that papers may be submitted to one journal after another before they are eventually published, they like the illusion that they are being offered first refusal, and authors are well advised to present their work in a fresh clean state, free from any marks which indicate that it has already been through other hands. Editors are not cheered by letters addressed to the wrong journal or by papers in a special format clearly intended for another journal; still less are they impressed by copies of correspondence from another journal, which has rejected the paper, recommending that the work be offered to them.

Where there is a choice of journals it is sensible to send the paper first to a journal showing a recent interest in the special area concerned. Editors will be pleased to see a paper developing further a field of interest or a paper contradicting previous published work. Editors are not usually pleased by papers which merely repeat work recently published in the same journal unless the subject is still highly controversial.

Most journals publish "notes for contributors" regularly; the author who wishes to please the editor will follow these to the letter. If the journal requires three copies of the manuscript, send three copies; if an abstract is required at the beginning, the paper should not be sent with a summary at the end instead. The references should be in the format required by the journal. It is worth making sure that the "notes for contributors" are current. The requirements for journals are changed from time to time as editors come and go. Even the address for submissions may change.

The *BMJ* publishes "guidelines for writing papers" regularly (most recently, 1989; **298**: 40.) Much of the advice given here is applicable to the preparation of manuscripts intended for any journal. In addition to the guidelines, several detailed checklists are published which guide referees, statisticians, and subeditors in their work. These are highly recommended reading for authors every time they prepare a manuscript.

Presentation of the text

Despite the wide availability of word processors, many manuscripts are poorly typed and badly set out. Simple faults create a bad impression. When it comes to editing the text the subeditor needs wide margins and true double spacing. This means that the distance between the lines on which the characters lie is twice the distance found in single spacing—not one and a half times the distance. The pages should be numbered, otherwise comments in referees' reports can be uninterpretable and, if the manuscript is dropped on the floor, the task of reconstructing it could prove too much for editorial patience. Editors dislike being sent a manuscript in the form of a zig-zag strip of fan-fold paper with the perforated strips still attached to the sides. Most of all they dislike the barely detectable output of a poor quality dot matrix printer operating in draft mode with a two year old ribbon.

Matters of style

Editors like simple direct English. Simplicity and brevity are admirable but only so far as the meaning remains clear. Papers must be capable of being understood by persons who have at least some interest in the subject but are not necessarily super-specialists (the editor himself often comes into this category). If the editor has received conflicting or only slightly enthusiastic referees' reports on a paper he will read it carefully to make his own assessment. If he finds it full of jargon and uninterpretable abbreviations he will probably give up and reject the paper, judging that the amount of editing work that would be required at a later stage would only be worth while if the article was otherwise outstanding.

Parts of the paper

Title—The title is a common blind spot for authors. It should be an honest but inviting indication of the contents. Some titles can be couched in the form of a question: "Do bananas heal venous ulcers?" In general, editors now discourage titles which make categorical statements: "Bananas heal venous ulcers".

Abstract—The abstract should be as informative as possible. The purpose and scope of the work should be indicated very briefly but the findings may be given in detail. The abstract should be capable of being understood on its own without reference to the paper and should not be treated as something equivalent to the trailer of a film in which the contents are suggested but the plot (and in particular the ending) is not divulged.

Introduction—This should provide no more than is essential for the average reader of the journal to understand why the study was undertaken. Except perhaps in the case of lengthy review articles the introduction is not an opportunity to display the depth of the author's scholarship or the breadth of his reading. Any references offered should be relevant and useful to other workers in the field.

Methods—Information in the methods section should be sufficient to allow other workers to repeat the study if necessary. When referring to previously reported methods, be sure that the method is exactly as previously reported or indicate departures from the original method and indicate in a few words what the method involves—this helps the non-expert reader. Statistical methods should be described, particularly where these are out of the mainstream.

Results—The results need to be given in detail, but the presentation need not be completely formal and bland. Surprising findings can be described as such and the reason for further measurements or analyses commented on in a logical narrative fashion. Where the results are best presented in a table they should not be repeated in detail in the text. Where summarising statistics have been used, it is essential to indicate what these are. Mean, median, standard deviation, standard error, range and other parameters all need to be specified. Editors particularly like 95% confidence limits. Missing data should be declared.

Discussion—The essence of the results can be summarised in a few words but the author should avoid repeating the whole of the results section. As well as comparing the work with relevant earlier work and discussing criticisms of both, there may be room for speculation. When speculating, be modest and brief and make it absolutely clear that you are speculating. It is comforting to finish an article with a rounding off sentence at the end rather than stopping in mid air. Every editor feels a sinking feeling, however, when offered the conclusion that "more work is required" and will usually put his pencil through any fond hope "that improved understanding of the underlying mechanisms of the disorder may lead ultimately to the development of a cure (or ... to its prevention)".

Figures—Figures should be drawn to professional standards. If graphs and similar technical figures in the target journal are redrawn as a matter of course (usually obvious as all such figures will have an identical style and identical lettering throughout the journal) it may be acceptable to have extremely clear draft versions. Mark the backs of figures clearly with name, figure number, and an indication of the top. Use a very soft pencil and do **not** use ball pen or felt tip pen. Even though the inks may seem to dry immediately they very commonly transfer on to the gelatin surface of adjacent prints over hours or days and the resulting damage can cause unnecessary stress and inconvenience for editors and authors alike. Figures require legends which will make them interpretable to the reader who merely skims the text. All abbreviations in the figure should be explained.

Tables—The first thing an editor looks at when he comes across a table is whether it is necessary. The second thing he looks at is whether the figures add up. Some editors can hardly resist checking tables even when reading other journals; checking becomes a sport and can deteriorate into an obsession. Simple errors are surprisingly common and result in an immediate drop in editorial confidence in the paper. Each table requires a heading which makes the contents clear to the reader who only skims through the text.

References—References should be perfect. When the editor first flicks through a newly submitted paper he will very probably look at a selection of the references. If he can detect one or two errors on the spot without referring to other sources he knows that indifferent care may have been taken with other parts of the paper and even with the work it reports. Most journals are not now able to check all references themselves and in the end the author must be relied on for accuracy. Mistakes with references are not taken lightly at any stage in the paper's processing. Editors warm to papers whose references are all referred to in the text (in the correct order) and are perfect to the last comma.

Revision—If an article is provisionally accepted on condition that certain points are dealt with satisfactorily, it helps the editor's work if the author submits an annotated list of points with an indication of how they have been dealt with. The numbering should match the list sent by the editor or referee. If only minor changes are requested and the editor has already edited the manuscript it may be unhelpful to retype or reprint the manuscript as this will result in the editor having to recheck the whole of the text to see that all of the changes have been incorporated. If changes are made to the text it pleases the editor if these are indicated in light pencil (or by highlighting on a photocopy). Any changes made by hand should be in pencil, rather than pen, and printed exquisitely clearly so that every letter is discernible.

Keep revisions to the proofs to an absolute minimum. Use only correct marks. Errors must of course be corrected, but this is not the moment for delicate adjustments to the phraseology or the insertion of a few more results or references.

Communicating with the editor

Editors are busy people. Most specialist journals are edited by part time editors who have normal, full time, clinical or academic commitments. It is easy for authors to forget that the editor of a journal might be handling 100 or 200 papers at various stages of assessment or preparation. Probably the most effective way of getting an editor's back up is to contact him or her directly by telephone and engage in urgent pleading about a paper. It is almost always pointless as the wary editor will avoid making any undertaking until he has had time to consider the matter with the manuscript in his hand and after referring to correspondence and referees' reports. The telephone caller who is not the first or corresponding author, and who does not know who the first author is or the paper's reference number, and is even unsure of the exact title is jeopardising his or her paper's chances.

If an author has something to communicate he should write a short letter and should quote the **reference number** of the paper as well as giving its title and first author. This allows the editor to deal with the matter in the time he allocates to journal affairs and permits him to refer to points in the manuscript and to check on such things as previously agreed conditions for publication.

Authors quite commonly pester editors before submitting an article, asking questions such as whether it is likely to be suitable and whether it can be looked at especially rapidly if it is submitted. The editor's reaction is predictable: "Let us have a look at it and we will assess it in the usual way". Nothing is gained and, if anything, there is a risk that the editor will be irritated by the special pleading and consequently be less sympathetic.

If you think that your paper has been unjustly criticised and rejected it may be worth resubmitting it with a compact, quietly reasoned argument meeting the objections. It is sensible to revise it first so as to meet all of the reasonable criticisms. It is very inadvisable to write an abusive letter to the editor. Some authors reserve their best talents for invective of this sort but the end result is usually counterproductive: editors have long memories.

Commissioned articles

So far, pleasing the editor has been discussed as a sensible adjuvant to acceptance of an unsolicited paper. Most journals have plenty of submitted articles to choose from and the editor can reject papers, or refuse to publish unless certain conditions are met, without feeling any need to please the author. When an editor commissions an author to write an article for a journal (or a chapter for a book), however, the relationship is different. The editor in effect takes a gamble. He hopes that the author will perceive precisely what he has in mind and then prepare a high quality manuscript. If the author produces something which is of a disappointing standard or wide of the target, the editor knows that it will require a great deal of tact, time, and probably personal work on the manuscript to recover the position. It will be difficult for the editor to refuse to publish the paper outright. Pleasing the commissioning editor is a matter of (1) writing about the subject requested and not something similar, (2) writing at a level which is appropriate to the intended readership, (3) writing to the required length and, most important of all, (4) getting it in before the deadline.

Editors are human, and like everyone else they are heartened by a letter of thanks. A letter of praise will bring lasting editorial pleasure until it finally fades inside its frame.

Further reading

O'Connor M, Woodford F P. *Writing scientific papers in English*. London: Pitman Medical, 1978.
Lock S. *Thorne's better medical writing*. 2nd ed. London: Pitman Medical, 1977.

Prepare a Festschrift

GREG WILKINSON

The word Festschrift (German *fest*, festival; *schrift*, writings; Pl.
-en, -s) is commonly used to designate the volume of essays,
papers, and the like prepared by colleagues and friends as a tribute
to a scholar or savant on some special occasion—usually on reach-
ing a certain age, stage of career, retirement, or anniversary.
"Festschriften", as Gerd Buchdal says, "are for men who have put
their stamp on some branch of enquiry during a certain period of
time."[1] Although the first recorded use of the word in English was
in 1901, there is still no satisfactory English equivalent. The preparation of a Festschrift is most commonly undertaken in the
German speaking countries. Elsewhere, it is much less common,
more often a tribute to distinguished figures in the humanities and
the basic sciences than in medicine.

Until now there has been no generally accepted method of preparing a Festschrift: varieties differ considerably in form and content. The typical format is most often that of a special issue or
supplement of a learned journal, or of an obscure publication,
rarely read (except by the recipient) and destined for a neglected
library shelf. Many, if not most, examples of the genre, whether
emanating from the arts or sciences, emerge as no more than an
ephemeral medley of stale material, reminiscences, and anecdotes,
flavoured with flattering commentaries on the person concerned.

As a consequence, the task of preparing a Festschrift is often
perceived as a dutiful chore, a secular act of devotion designed to
give pleasure to the recipient but mainly heartache to the editors.
Too much effort surrounds the preparation and too little thought is
given to the purpose.

Accordingly, when my colleagues and I decided to embark on a
Festschrift for Professor Michael Shepherd, we decided to try and
construct a new model, one which would be original and constitute

an enduring work of academic scholarship in its own right, becoming an essential point of reference for the subject, and indicating new points of departure. The theme of such a Festschrift should ideally derive from the work of its dedicatee and in this case the theory and practice of the epidemiological approach to mental disorder was the obvious choice.[2] Until his retirement in October 1988 Professor Shepherd had held the chair of epidemiological psychiatry at the Institute of Psychiatry, the first of its kind in the world, and his own contributions have played a major part in indicating the scope of the field as it has emerged over a generation.

Genesis

The proposed volume was conceived as bringing together theory, experiment, and practical applications and was subdivided into six sections. The first, a brief introduction by the editors, outlined the purpose and scope of the work; the second was concerned with the scientific principles which underpin epidemiological investigations; the third was divided into three subsections, each of which concerned a particular area of enquiry within the general field; the fourth was concerned with the evaluation of psychiatric intervention, and was divided into subsections which focused, respectively, on the organisation of services and the assessment of specific treatments; the fifth provided international perspectives; and the sixth and final section gave a personal overview of Professor Shepherd's achievement.

To represent the range and nature of his influence, our aim was to bring together a group of colleagues who had had professional association with him at a number of levels. We then contacted a likely publisher, sending a detailed outline, including details of chapters and the names of prospective contributors. Financial and administrative aspects of publication were also dealt with at this stage.

Next, we invited an international group of around 40 distinguished clinicians and academics to contribute, giving them specific instructions, an example of which runs as follows:

> We are inviting you to write a chapter for the section on the scientific principles which underpin epidemiology, and would like you to discuss the relevance and importance of statistical understanding for the prosecution of research in epidemio-

logical psychiatry. We expect that each chapter will be about 5000 words long, and we hope to deliver the manuscript to the publisher in nine months time.

The invitation had to be qualified as follows:

> Although you will receive a free copy of the book, the publishers regret that in view of the large number of contributors, it will not be possible to offer a fee. We also regret this, but hope that you will none the less agree to contribute. If, as we hope, you do agree to participate, we will write to you again soon to clarify the nature of your contribution and the details of the publishing schedule.

We sent contributors precise guidelines, including a copy of the most relevant parts of the publisher's house style booklet and a full list of contents and contributors. We took care to give individual guidance on possible areas of overlap. We emphasised that we did not want irrelevant or anecdotal mention of Professor Shepherd in the text, though his work could be referred to in a conventional manner when necessary.

On course

There were few early complications. One of our contributors had to drop out but we quickly found a replacement. Later, there were more thorny problems: one contributor's instructions had evidently not been explicit enough; one wrote twice as many words as requested, so the typescript was returned; another insisted on having numerous references printed in an unconventional style; a European contributor, though fluent in English, submitted his work in native tongue. Duplication and redundancy were minimal. Several figures and tables needed to be redrawn for publication, and a few contributors had changed address and title.

In the course of time we increased the number of chapters and contributors as our ideas crystallised. We drafted introductions to the various sections of the volume—a relatively easy task as instructions to authors were so specific. Close to the stated deadline we wrote an encouraging letter of inquiry to far flung contributors and tackled those closer to home more robustly.

As anticipated, the material was submitted to the publisher six months over schedule. The planned 140 000 words had snowballed

THE SCOPE OF EPIDEMIOLOGICAL PSYCHIATRY

*Essays in Honour of
Michael Shepherd*

Edited by
PAUL WILLIAMS
GREG WILKINSON
KENNETH RAWNSLEY

ROUTLEDGE
London and New York

to reach 250 000. The subeditor's textual queries appeared with, as usual, many peculiar and unexpected errors to correct or clarify. There were abundant problems with references. Total commitment and lengthy national and international telephone calls with contributors were required, thus ensuring that all difficulties were dealt with within the allotted week. Shortly afterwards proofs arrived: because of time constraints we decided not to send them to authors. The main finding—a quarter of one chapter had been duplicated. We also found it particularly important to check contributors' names, titles, and addresses, the lists of contents and contributors, chapter headings and index. Lastly, we provided the publisher with an (approved) photograph of our subject for a discrete position on the dust-jacket.

The book, some 550 pages in length, was officially launched at the beginning of 1989 and has been well reviewed.[3][4] After publication one contributor was temporarily aggrieved because a portion of her submission was edited without consent; another was wounded because his recently elevated status had not been acknowledged; a surname had been misspelt in the list of contents. Several colleagues complained that they had not been invited to contribute.

Finally, to celebrate the publication we organised a dinner for contributors and publisher, at which Michael Shepherd was presented with a leather-bound copy of the Festschrift. A photograph was taken to mark the occasion and was sent as a souvenir to everyone concerned.

Unexpectedly, the form of our Festschrift has already attracted some attention as a possible model for tributes of this type. We have come to the opinion that its construction might provide a more appropriate and more permanent accolade on such occasions. In view of the associations of the word Festschrift, however, perhaps another word is needed. We have wondered about Festschrift or tributary volume. Other suggestions would be welcomed.

References

1 Buchdahl G. Nagel's message. *Nature* 1971; **231**: 399.
2 Williams P, Wilkinson G, Rawnsley K. *The scope of epidemiological psychiatry. Essays in honour of Michael Shepherd.* London: Routledge, 1989.
3 Johnstone E C. The scope of epidemiological psychiatry. *Lancet* 1989; **i**: 588.
4 Charlton B. Wider still and wider. . . . *Br Med J* 1989; **298**: 1193–4.

Get publicity

PAMELA TAYLOR

When it comes to getting publicity, thinking through the consequences before you take any public action can make all the difference between sensationalised press headlines, which alienate your colleagues and alarm your patients, and sensible reports which accurately set out your position.

Perhaps the most difficult aspect of generating publicity is recognising yourself what is newsworthy and what is not. Achieving publicity means simplifying a complex issue and making it readily understandable by the public. This is not trivialising the subject; it is the art of communicating with the public on their own terms, just as an individual doctor should be able to communicate with a patient on that patient's terms.

Medicine is known as a "must subject" for the press; they must cover it. The column inches, radio, and television time devoted to health issues are still increasing, and that is because health issues have all the ingredients the public loves: life and death, human interest, and, crucially, health is recognised as being relevant to each one of us.

The first essential step in achieving publicity is to find a "peg". A peg is journalese for something to hang the story on; that means an action or event taking place now. You and your colleauges may have complained about funding for months but the peg for the newspaper stories would be your letter of protest today to the local Member of Parliament.

While the politics of the NHS hits the headlines, remember that scientific information, too, can be made accessible to the public. When the Army Blood Supply Depot devised a new freezing technique for prolonging the storage of blood the *Standard* headline proclaimed, "A Chilling Success for Vampires" over a story which clearly explained the techniques and, importantly for the readers, told of the future relevance to civilian hospitals and saving lives in the NHS.

Writing to the Press

One of the least traumatic forays into the media can be achieved by writing a letter for publication in a newspaper.

Your letter can be in response to an article already printed, but there is nothing to stop you from writing on any aspect of health which you believe will be of interest to the newspaper's readers. You may want to use your local press to encourage women to come forward for cervical screening or you may want to use the national press to alert the public to the problems caused by split site facilities and anaesthetic cover. Either way, the rules are the same.

- Keep your letter short, particularly if you are writing to one of the tabloids.
- Avoid jargon.
- Make your letter relevant to the readers of the particular newspaper.
- Before you send the letter, inform your colleagues and double-check your facts.

Ring the Letters page and tell them your letter is on its way. Keep a copy. Sometimes the Letters editor will ring you and negotiate some cuts to fit your contribution on to the page; sometimes a butchered version is printed without any consultation. Chase them up if nothing appears in print, and don't be afraid to send your letter to a second newspaper, provided it is relevant to its readers, if the first one decides against publication.

Local radio

There are countless air-time hours to be filled, and the public loves to hear about health issues. If you feel brave enough the opportunities are there for you to put your message out on the airwaves.

All you have to do is to ring the local radio station, explain what you would like to say, and ask them if they are interested. You must have something newsworthy to say, but you can rely on the judgment of the local radio staff to tell you whether you are worth interviewing. Initially it is as simple as that.

What might they be interested in? National news stories often have a local news aspect which can be highlighted. Smoking is regularly in the national news and many doctors are successful in persuading their local radio stations to run a local interview on young people and smoking, or a phone-in for people wanting to give up.

Now comes the more difficult part—the interview itself. Draw up a check list of questions to ask the interviewer in advance.

- When is the interview?
- What programme will it be broadcast on?
- Will it be live or recorded?
- What will be the venue—surgery, hospital, or studio?
- Will others also be interviewed—will their views be opposed to yours?

Then take time to prepare yourself. Write down a maximum of five key points you want to put over to the audience. Make them positive and informative points, and stick to them. During the interview, listen to the question then select one of your key points in response. If the first question is very far removed from any of your key points simply say "I think it's important to say right at the start that ..." then introduce one of the points you planned to make. So long as your point is positive and relevant, the interviewer will allow this.

If you are a success they may offer you a regular radio doctor slot. But that is another skill and another story.

Producing a press statement

The easiest way to inform several journalists about your views is to write a press statement and send it to them all. A good press statement is simply written, avoiding hyperbole, and structured to answer the questions—who? what? when? where? and why?

What could possibly be of interest to the press that is of help to you? Work involving the community is a sure winner. A joint plea by hospital doctors and GPs for adequate meal services and improved home care for elderly patients discharged from hospitals would be of interest to the press, radio, and probably regional television. A booklet available to the public on healthy eating, new measures to reach ethnic minorities, or a letter to your MP on local

NHS funding would all make suitable material for a press statement.

(i) The opening paragraph of your press statement should sum up the whole story:

Blanktown's GPs and hospital doctors have today written to their MP protesting that local cuts in health service financing are threatening the standards of services to patients.

(ii) The second paragraph should contain details to expand on the opening paragraph. In this example details of services to be cut could be given.

(iii) The final paragraph can be in the form of a quote where opinions can be expressed:

Dr Joan Smith commented, "We are concerned for our patients..."

(iv) Make sure there is a contact name and a telephone number, or numbers, so journalists with queries can ring for further information at any time.

Consult your colleagues when necessary; it is no use jumping up and down about a funding crisis if the press hear from one of your colleagues that he has no idea what you are on about. Send the press statement, either in the post or, ideally, by hand, addressed to the News Desk, unless you have the name of a particular journalist. It helps if it arrives early in the day so the journalists have time to work on it. Ring them and offer to help whoever has been allocated to write a story based on the statement. This often helps to establish the vital fact that your statement has not even progressed beyond the front reception desk.

Press conferences

The information you want to put across to the media may be too complex to be contained in a press statement. What sort of subject would persuade the journalist to come and listen to you?

The opening of a new hospital or wing is an obvious, though rare, opportunity. The press would be quite happy, though, to cover the provision of new facilities, particularly if there is some impressive equipment they can photograph. Closures and cuts in services are big news, too.

Press conferences announcing fund raising stunts, deputations, and organised protests are the stuff of local paper front page headlines. When doctors in Scotland took to the streets in their white coats to protest at the building of a factory to manufacture chewing tobacco, the press conference and march made headlines in the United Kingdom. Organising a press conference needs:

- a time, probably in the morning;
- a place with a top table and chairs facing for the press;
- invitations to the press, either written or telephoned;
- two or three people to give the press conference.

Press visits

Why not open the doors and allow the Press in? Such an invitation can be disarming, particularly if you have been on the receiving end of some bad publicity. The Press would respond to an invitation to see a deputising service at work, or to view the poor accommodation for junior hospital doctors. Having the Press tramping around disrupting the working routine and accosting patients is what you want to avoid. So a successful open day needs to be planned:

- map out a timetable;
- concentrate on positive points to put across;
- consult internally;
- involve all relevant staff;
- obtain permission from any patients who may be involved;
- hold a dress rehearsal;
- organise the catering (coffee on arrival, with sandwiches and soft drinks for lunch are quite sufficient).

Ensure that everyone who may come into contact with the Press during the visit is well briefed on what to say and, just as important, what not to say. An apparently helpful expansion by one doctor on another's views can appear in the press as, "local doctors split on the best way to treat...".

Television

Television is all about interesting pictures. A row of doctors sitting in the postgraduate centre speaking at a press conference does not afford television the most exciting scenes. If your message is interesting enough, though, producers will want to interview you, but they really want more than what they term "talking heads": they want action.

A well organised picture opportunity often makes all the difference between no TV interest and hitting the headlines. Even tired old messages can be brought to life.

You will not receive television coverage for warnings about road traffic accidents, but lit candles depicting the number of avoidable deaths should ensure that your message is televised. Similarly, financial wrangling over the threatened closure of a special baby care unit is unlikely material for peak time viewing, but a gathering of mothers with their babies who have been successfully treated by the unit should make it on to the screens.

Television pictures take time to organise. Filming is expensive and camera crews' time planned carefully. Make sure you:

- ring the television news intake desk two or three days beforehand;
- discuss in advance the sort of pictures they will want to take;
- discuss timing (you do not want to miss the lunchtime news bulletins).
- Will they want to interview someone in addition to taking general pictures; if so who, where, and when?

Surviving a television interview means acting larger than life. Look interested in what you are saying and be positive. And watch your language. Avoid saying "patient care" when you can say "the care of patients" and "working beyond their contractual obligations" when you can say "doctors and nurses are working very hard". Many doctors on television alienate the viewers when they hide behind such medical clichés.

You will be on air for a few moments, so talk in headlines rather than meticulously building up to a point. Dump most of the information you have in your mind and just concentrate on the major points you want the public to know about. Increasingly, news editors are looking for "sound bites". They want one illustrative sentence which they can pull out of the recording and use up front in the news story, with perhaps a subsidiary sentence slotted into the same news item towards the end.

Using publicity

Publicity is a powerful tool and should be used thoughtfully. At worst it can cause damage and real distress, but used wisely it can help bring about real change for the better.

Apply for charitable status

MAURICE SLEVIN, PATSY RYAN

Creating a unique information service for patients with cancer wasn't Dr Vicky Clement-Jones's only unusual achievement when she founded the British Association of Cancer United Patients (BACUP) in 1984; she also gave a new twist to the old adage "charity begins at home," as most of the groundwork was done from her home in London while she was convalescing after treatment for advanced ovarian cancer. As her plans gathered momentum and she and willing colleagues were caught up in the frantic merry go round of raising funds, forging contacts, and generally securing a place in the hearts (and pockets) of philanthropic money makers the advantages of acquiring charitable status beckoned invitingly.

Vicky seized all opportunities with characteristic spirit and vigour, and her inspiring enthusiasm (coupled with a sense of true urgency as her prognosis was uncertain) led to the association being registered as a charity in just three days. The year of 1984 certainly had its fair share of unique achievements.

Pros and cons

The first question a potential charity crusader should ask, uncharitably enough, is, "How will charitable status give my plans the edge?" The solution comes from objectively weighing up the pros and cons and banishing Dickensian overtones of the term charity.

The major advantage is financial. The great British public is reassured by the respectability of a registered charity number when being persuaded to part with hard earned cash. Even if you don't envisage rattling collecting tins at Saturday afternoon shoppers, when you are appealing to benevolent businesses and charitable foundations the magic number proves an effective open sesame to their coffers. More pragmatically, registered charities are automatically entitled to 50% rates relief on premises—some generous local authorities even offer 100% relief. Some useful exemptions from value added tax and stamp duty relax tense purse strings, and opportunities for donations free of tax gild the carrot to tempt valuable regular donors.

The commonest drawbacks to attaining charitable status are the strict legal limitations imposed on political and campaigning activities. This is sensitive territory, and if planning to venture into it you would be well advised to have the guiding hand of a good lawyer at your elbow.

Your best guide is generally a solicitor experienced in all aspects of forming charities. The increasingly complex charity laws are a specialist subject, and experts tend to be thin on the ground. Your willing regular solicitor, however, could do the job ably assisted by the Charity Law Advisory Service for Solicitors. This is a service to which lawyers can turn for practical and expert help with charity law. The National Council for Voluntary Organisations can also give legal advice and supply model constitutions for budding founders of a charity.

Paths paved with charitable intentions

Since 1891 British law has recognised only four distinct categories of charitable purposes. So, unfortunately, however worthy the intentions of your future organisation the law (and therefore charitable status) will remain impervious unless you can slot your aims neatly into one of those four categories.

Categories of charitable purposes

- Relief of poverty
- Advancement of education
- Advancement of religion
- Specific other purposes beneficial to the community

Hand in hand with advice from your legal mentor on how to satisfy the legal criteria of these categories should go the principle of saving time and resources: "Never reinvent the wheel." When BACUP had little more substance than a pipe dream Vicky embarked on a fact finding mission to the United States National Cancer Institute. She returned with two suitcases crammed full of invaluable anecdotal advice and experience. Avoiding the mistakes and using the successes of others serve as a whetstone to sharpen your aims and speed your progress.

Building the empire

Basically, the constitution of a charity (or governing instrument, to use the legally accurate term) should define the purposes and powers of the organisation and agree the means of achieving them to avoid disputes at a later date. As this worthy document is also one of the chief components of the application for registration as a charity it is worth while investing time and effort to make it absolutely accurate.

Fortunately, plagiarism of a model constitution is acceptable—even advisable—if the chosen model fits your aims like a glove. If original thought is called for, however, the chief architect must remember that the formal constitution is the bricks and mortar of a charity. It must be sturdily constructed to withstand collapsing into rubble at the first knock.

Once the basic constitutional foundations have been laid allow your lawyer to guide you through the plethora of legal formats available to use as your charity's floor plans. For instance, will you form an unincorporated organisation (a trust, for example) or an incorporated organisation (such as a company limited by guarantee)? Do you visualise running a benevolent dictatorship from central headquarters or will you opt for regional centres each with a degree of autonomy? The alternatives are legion, and the consequences of finalising flawed plans can be disastrous for a fledgling charity. Expert legal advice is probably mandatory.

Every empire needs its pillars; every charity needs its trustees or directors. These guardians of the charity's assets and aims are invested with the general control and management of the charity. In a nutshell, they exercise full sway over what the charity does and how it does it. So, although selecting international superstars may add a certain cachet to your organisation, if the candidates can boast appropriate professional skills to back up their superstardom so much the better. If after appointing trustees or directors, however, you have a couple of left over "unqualified" superstars waiting in the wings endow them with the honorary title of patron. This is an economical way of using their names and backing without entangling them in the running of the charity.

The grand launch

The blessing of new organisations with charitable status has been firmly in the hands of the Charity Commissioners for England and Wales since 1960, since when all charities have been required by law to register with this body. After receiving your application the commissioners will carefully study your constitution and a statement of your proposed activities before bestowing charitable status on you—or not, as the case may be.

If at first you don't succeed apply, apply again. Your solicitor can argue your case with the commissioners or you may need to alter some details of your constitution to satisfy dissenters. If necessary an expert solicitor may even be able to prove that the commissioners' objections have no legal basis. Remember, any group is basically eligible to register as a charity provided it is willing to conform to current interpretations of the four categories of charitable purposes. Be flexible and well informed. Don't be browbeaten by long delays and minor misunderstandings. Finally, repeat this mantra at regular intervals: "Rome wasn't built in a day."

Once the charity commissioners have approved your constitution, adopt it formally and you will be allocated your registered charity number to print reassuringly on stationery and fundraising material, with a statement confirming your charitable status. In return, you must supply the commissioners with yearly audited accounts of your financial state of health and get their approval for any planned fundamental changes in the charity's constitution.

Taking it all into consideration, and despite the restrictions imposed by law, founding a charity is the perfect chance of a lifetime to etch your own lasting design on history's slate. Perhaps Vicky's example of starting BACUP with just one person and £32 000 raised from friends and patients will be an inspiration to others to take the plunge into the charity pool. Now, four years later, her legacy to the nation is helping 100 patients with cancer each day, employing over 20 professional staff, and working to meet an annual budget which, in the near future will approach £1 000 000.

Further reading

Phillips A. *Charitable status, a practical handbook.* 3rd ed. London: InterChange Books, 1988.

Survive a dinner

CLIFFORD HAWKINS

Public dinners provide an occupational hazard for VIPs such as presidents of royal colleges, vice chancellors, deans, and others. The risks to health are minimal; obesity, bowel upset, and, rarely, hepatitis (a severe outbreak of this followed a dinner held at an ancient medical society in London). Formerly there were dangers. Max Beerbohm described 'how, in the fifteenth century, some members of the renowned family of Borgia laid down rare poisons in their cellars with as much thought as they gave to their vintage wine. An invitation to dine at the Palazzio Borgese was regarded as the highest social honour, but whereas the snobbish Roman might say in an offhand way "I am dining with the Borgias tonight," it is unlikely that he would say "I dined last night with the Borgias."[1] I will consider here, however, the irritations and frustrations that afflict habitués of dinners, especially the problems of the after dinner speaker.

The reception

A hardened and distinguished diner described the reception as the preprandial cacophony. People speak louder and louder to compete with the general clamour, and this makes communication more and more difficult. An ear trumpet would be useful, or perhaps a gong should sound periodically to proclaim a moment of silence so that conversation could start again quietly.

Joining the reception when it is in full swing presents no problem on home territory. When it is elsewhere the usual advice is to obtain a drink and then approach someone you know or think you recognise. This can be risky. The story goes that a guest went up to a woman whose appearance seemed familiar and the following conversation took place:

"How is your father these days?"
"Oh, he has died."
"I'm so sorry; when was this?"
"Thirty five years ago."
"Tell me about your brother."
"I haven't got a brother."
"Sorry, I meant your sister."
"Oh, she's still on the throne."

Small talk does not come easily to everyone, and the energy drain of light polite conversation with strangers in a confined space can be considerable. Moreover, the impaction of bodies makes it difficult to extricate yourself and to circulate, so that you are sometimes rooted to the spot until every topic has been exhausted—and there is seldom anywhere to sit down. The background chatter makes it difficult to catch the name of those to whom you are introduced, and it is easy to forget this when passing on the introduction to another: the legible lapel label is a blessing. Forgetting the names or appointments of those met only occasionally is easy, especially for public figures, who meet so many. The cliché "I remember your face but have forgotten your name," which is usually true, is preferable to "I remember your name but have forgotten your face." Americans help by introducing themselves with a brief biographical sketch, such as, "I'm Casper Fitzwater, married with four children, live in Boston, and my special interest is pneukalgiography."

Background music creates a relaxed ambience. But it should be gentle chamber music and not (as happened at a reception I attended last year) a boisterous wind ensemble that obliterates human voices. The musicians, perhaps from the local music college, must be told that guests may not take any notice of them. A few chairs should be provided for those who wish to listen or just to sit down.

Time spent in reconnaissance is seldom wasted: studying the seating plan and, when necessary, finding out about neighbouring diners. When there is no plan the temptation to join colleagues whom you see regularly is best avoided: either seek out friends who are otherwise seldom seen or take pot luck and sit anywhere. Wine, if not included in the cost of the dinner, should be ordered early; once the dinner has started the busy staff will be difficult to corner—a point that explains the epitaph suggested for the tombstone of a waiter: "God finally caught his eye."

At the dinner

A seating plan is essential for the top or high table, otherwise diners will shun it, and unless tables are clearly marked some diners may be wandering around when the VIPs come in or as grace is starting. Talking is limited at the top table, where no one sits opposite; sometimes long tables are too wide for conversation. Separate round tables are increasingly a feature of public dinners and avoid the isolation of the top table; but vision should not be obscured by a bowl of flowers. Isolation is also caused by empty places, and doctors who accept invitations but fail to turn up and give no warning or apology are a particular annoyance to pharmaceutical firms that provide hospitality at medical meetings.

Whether or not grace will be said must be made clear, otherwise diners may be caught halfway between sitting and standing. Some think that grace is an outmoded ritual, and a wit considered it odd that the Lord should be thanked before you know what has been provided. Latin graces beginning with "Benedicite" are seldom understood, and several lines of Latin are hardly more than an ego trip for the speaker. A fundamentalist Christian grace seems inappropriate in our multiracial society. A suitable form of words may be "Let us give thanks for the food and drink we are about to receive and spare a thought for those who are less fortunate"—not that a thought alone may be of much help to them.

Dinners are often remembered by the company that has been enjoyed. Prowess in conversation varies; a cynic said that a gossip talks about others, a bore talks about himself, and a brilliant conversationalist talks about you. The evening can be spoiled if the diner never sees other than the back of his or her neighbour, who is concerned with two or three others interested only in shop talk. On the other hand, however interesting an enthusiastic talker may be, it is helpful if he or she, like Macaulay, "has occasional flashes of silence that make his conversation delightful,"[2] as one object of a dinner is to enjoy the food. Conducting a dual discussion with someone on each side could be risky: choking might be caused by attempting to answer a question with a mouthful of, perhaps, sherry trifle garnished with brandy snaps, as no one may be capable of performing the Heimlich manoeuvre.

The food

Meals have improved over the past 20 years owing to deep

freezers and microwave ovens. But public dinners are not for the gourmet for, as Rose Macaulay wrote, "another sad comestive truth is that the best foods are the products of infinite and wearying trouble,"[3] and preparing them is impossible when catering for large numbers. It is difficult to please everyone, and some diners may be vegetarians or have religious taboos. Tastes vary; some like beef well done and others prefer it rare. Lamb was once a safe choice, but the vogue now is to have it underdone. Many foods spoil if reheated and go off if kept warm; casseroles such as coq au vin and beef stroganoff are an exception. Thin tasteless slices of electrically cut meat steeped in lukewarm gravy fail to tempt the appetite, and portions are often too large for the average eater. Those brought up to leave the plate clean feel guilty, but others reared in the affluent society leave food uneaten without feeling this.

Slap handed service is a rare hazard. On one occasion the guest speaker and the wife of a distinguished guest were both doused with soup; if this happens the head waiter apologises and the caterers' insurance puts right the damage.

The drink

Gone are the days when some, having wined well, would slump into their cars, somewhat inebriated, and drive home. Such behaviour no longer provides a macho image and is socially unacceptable. Wine that "maketh glad the heart of man" has to be taken in moderation and—what sacrilege—orange juice instead of port if you are driving home. Happy is the diner whose spouse remains teetotal for the evening and can act as chauffeur. Water, which as Mark Twain said, "taken in moderation cannot hurt anybody," should be on the table and not need to be asked for.

The essential interval after the royal toast allows a visit to the "comfort station." Anyone intent on smoking should ask whether any at the table are misocapnists, especially now that many more hate tobacco smoke because of the possible risk of passive smoking.

Listening to after dinner speaking

After dinner speeches can make or mar the evening.[4] Sometimes, when the wine and good food have created a climax of conviviality, a dull silence falls and the jovial atmosphere disappears as the speaker delivers a speech that has cost him restless nights in its conception and anorexia during the meal. Occasionally the victim makes a speech that holds the audience in interest and mirth—a fine ending to a meal and a good prelude to the rest of the evening. If speeches are dull and long the diners get stuck in their places and opposite the same old faces.[5] They are a captive audience and there is no time limit or chairman to call a halt. About eight minutes is the customary length, but 20 minutes or more may be expected from the solo guest speaker. There is a good case for limiting speeches to two.

Listeners expect to be amused, but humour is not everyone's forte. One result is a forced funniness and, at the worst, a series of worn out and irrelevant jokes, some of which may be risqué and embarrass the audience. Listing the top 10 phrases used by speakers, Miles Kingston gave the winning phrase as "In this context, I am reminded of the story . . . "; others were "An anecdote comes to mind . . . ," and "Which reminds me of an incident. . . ." He suggested that an after dinner speech should be brief, witty, and clean.[6] Jokes are useful to illustrate serious ideas, and humour should be natural, original and unpredictable, if possible, and appropriate to the audience. Shakespeare understood this: as Viola remarked in *Twelfth Night*, "This fellow's wise enough to play the fool and to do that well craves a kind of wit: he must observe their mood on whom he jests, the quality of persons, and the time." Excellent speeches can be made without a single joke, the best being casually witty, although basically serious.

Some speeches put the listeners to sleep. This can happen at the annual dinner when the chairman decides that he has to report on "the state of the union" and dwells endlessly on unnecessary details of the year's activities. Members have no time to circulate; they slink home exhausted to bed. Sir Francis Walshe wrote, "the toast of the guests is always the nadir of after dinner oratory. It would be a healthy custom if every proposer of this toast who started on the *Who's Who* tack were swiftly and silently removed from the room. Nothing else will save us from these unimaginative bores."[7]

Plight of the after dinner speaker

Few leap with joy when they receive an invitation to "say a few words after dinner." A colleague who lectures in this country and abroad was concerned at having to speak at a formal dinner after he had received an honorary degree from a university. A distinguished professor of medicine stated that after dinner speeches should be given by those who are gifted and that others should never speak, but there were some like himself who are required to speak and need advice. A cabinet minister who appears regularly on television said that he likes going to dinners except when he has to speak, although he is pleased to get up at any time and talk about politics.

Enjoyment of the dinner may be spoiled by apprehension. No trial has been done on the effect of β blockers. Alcohol helps, but too much is disastrous: speak first and drink later. The call to begin is especially alarming when announced by the thunderous decibels of the crimson jacketed toastmaster on a formal occasion. The speaker stands alone, a pinnacle in a sea of expectant faces, and may have to begin while waitresses flit around serving coffee or noises come from the adjacent kitchen.

Some believe that good speaking, like good writing, comes easily, but for most mortals hard work is needed for both. This certainly applied to Richard Asher, physician, writer, and scintillating talker. I once looked forward to enjoying the company of Dr T F Fox, a distinguished former editor of the *Lancet*, whom I had arranged to entertain before his speech at our annual medical society dinner, but he apologised and spent those 30 minutes or more with his head buried in his notes. Yet when he spoke it seemed as if it were an impromptu talk. Mark Twain stated that it usually takes no more than three weeks to prepare an impromptu speech. No doubt the high standard of many of the speeches given today is due to a similar devotion.

The ideal speech should be friendly, slightly discursive, appropriate for the occasion, and to some extent light hearted to avoid destroying postprandial conviviality. Lack of confidence is an asset, and the best speakers get nervous beforehand; the worst speeches are given by those who suffer from overconfidence and enjoy listening to the cadence of their own voices.

Hazards of speaking

Whether invited as a guest speaker because of his or her distinction or because of the office held the speaker is likely to address an amiable and sympathetic audience whose receptivity has been increased by the food and wine. A modest start endears the speaker to the audience and is usually sincere but must be put carefully. A risky way of invoking the "weakness of the chosen vessel" theme is to begin with "Goodness only knows why I am making this speech" or "No doubt you must be hoping that the old bore will shut up and sit down." The morale of even the most self confident person will be disturbed if this is received in sullen silence, perhaps broken by a few mutterings of "Hear, hear" instead of laughter.

Notes are useful for moral support and as reminders in case of speaker's block. They can be written on record cards, kept as simple as possible, made legible (as they will be further away than the customary lectern), and held loosely together (by treasury tags or rings) in case they are dropped. The cards can be placed unobtrusively behind a bowl of flowers or the wine glasses, or held in the hand if small. Even Sir Derrick Dunlop, a most polished and experienced speaker, believed in having notes; once he was delivering a memorial address in Edinburgh cathedral without notes when he had the appalling experience of his mind suddenly going blank.

Worst of all is, as Girdwood aptly described, is to be asked to speak off the cuff without warning.[8] And nearly as bad is to be the last speaker. To be called on at a very late hour after several long speeches have been made is a nightmare. As Norman Birkett, the distinguished judge, wrote, "Many of the diners are hurrying from the hall before the speaker rises so that they can catch the last train home, and there is a general air of having-had-enough-speaking-for-one-night abroad." He quoted the solution of another judge, Lord Hewart, to whom this happened. He told his audience that, fearing this situation, he had prepared two speeches in order to meet any eventuality. One speech was a short speech, the other was a little longer, and he was considering what he should do. After keeping the listeners in suspense for some moments he announced that he had decided to give them both; here the audience uttered a long, collective sigh. He then went on, "I will begin with the short one which was 'Thank you,' and I will also give you the longer one, which was 'Thank you very much.'" He then sat down to the longest applause of the evening.[9]

Finally there comes the vote of thanks, which should be limited to a minute or two. It is pleasant to hear a few flattering words but disheartening when the speaker goes off on his or her own tack and forgets to mention your effort—or starts on a long recap of the speech just heard. Every speaker should end before the attention of the listeners has started to wane.

Needs of the speaker

A good organiser appreciates the needs of the speaker and briefs him or her clearly about the occasion: whether the audience will be medical, or mixed with lay people and spouses, whether there will be the one speech or several, and whether a toast will be required. Most speakers are looked after well, but lapses are possible.[10]

The speaker should be cosseted: recognised on arrival instead of having to force a way through the crowded reception to find the host and given a good send off. Even professional after dinner speakers have their trials and tribulations. Basil Boothroyd wrote, "He enters their life for an hour, filling a speaker shaped space like a fairground cut-out. How should they guess that it's not an hour but a week out of his life, mostly with bad nights and delirious mutterings? Why, when he's gone, should they give him another thought, as he lurks at a cabless Euston or sprints for the Cincinnati plane?"[11]

References

1   Max Beerbohm. The incomparable Max. In: Roberts S C, ed. *Hosts and guests.* London: Heinemann, 1962; **248**:244–57.
2   Holland S. *A memoir of the Reverend Sydney Smith by his daughter, Lady Holland.* Vol 1, 2nd ed. London: Longmans, 1855; 366.
3   Macaulay R. Personal pleasures. In: Ray C, ed. *The gourmet's companion.* London: Eyre and Spottiswoode, 1963; 323.
4   Hawkins C, After-dinner speaking. *Br Med J* 1988; **297**: 1693–5.
5   Anonymous. After dinner [Editorial]. *Br Med J* 1958; **ii**: 904.
6   Kington M. *Independent* June 30 1987; 14 (col 1).
7   Walshe F. After dinner. *Br Med J* 1958; **ii**: 1039–40.
8   Girdwood R H. Performances that went wrong. *Br Med J* 1987; **295**: 1668–90.
9   Birkett N. On saying a few words after dinner. *Punch* November 2 1959: 12–4.
10 Lock S. Nice people with no manners. *Br Med J* 1978; **ii**: 1774–5.
11 Boothroyd B. *Accustomed as I am: the loneliness of the long-distance speaker.* London: Allen & Unwin, 1975: 12.

Look after a visiting speaker

PATRICK HOYTE

In the course of my work for a medical defence organisation I have lectured around 150 times over the past five years. Some of the audiences have been non-medical—for example, health economists, nurses, administrators—and some have been students, but most of my speaking engagements have been to medical audiences of one sort or another—postgraduate societies, BMA divisions, courses for trainee general practitioners, courses for family planners, specialist symposia.

Anyone accustomed to this sort of regular lecture circuit will be well aware of the immense variety of venue, host, and hospitality. While the venue itself may not be too important, provided one has been given the information to find it at all, some standards of hospitality leave a lot to be desired; although I am happy to say that the really bad examples are very much in the minority.

Two disasters . . .

In February 1988 I was asked to speak to an evening meeting of a medical group in the midlands. I specifically asked the organiser for a slide projector to be made available and went ahead with travel arrangements including a hotel booking. When I arrived at the venue after a 60 mile drive, I found that the meeting had been cancelled because there was no projector and that the organiser had sent only a deputy to apologise. Given an audience I could, of course, have spoken perfectly well without visual aids, but was not consulted, although the cancellation had only been announced earlier the same day. No offer of a lecture fee, travelling, or subsistence expenses was made.

Six months previously I had spoken to a specialist symposium at a major teaching hospital. There was no one to meet me when I arrived as the organiser was listening to the previous speaker. The promised meal was almost all gone and was in any case cold, and there were no clean plates, cups, or cutlery. The previous speaker exceeded his time by about half an hour, and it was another 20 minutes before the visual aids (in this case a video recorder) could be made to work for my own presentation. Even though it was an evening meeting, no lecture fee or travelling expenses were paid.

. . . and a triumph

The following evening I was contracted to speak to a post-graduate society in Lincolnshire. A map of the town and of the hospital were sent to me and a parking space was set aside; the organiser and the postgraduate secretary were waiting in the door-way to greet me; I was offered an excellent meal and choice of drinks and placed with pleasant company; I was even shown the "gents" without having to ask. The meeting itself went well, the large audience asked a lot of stimulating questions, and informal discussion went on for some time after that. A lecture fee and travelling expenses were paid and I received a pleasant "thank you letter" from the postgraduate tutor.

Do's and don'ts

The examples I have given are clearly opposite ends of a large spectrum, but I do not doubt that the "disaster" organisers would have been quick to criticise if my presentations had attained only the standards they apparently set for themselves. I therefore put forward the following slightly tongue-in-cheek aide mémoire for the benefit of those who wish to invite visiting speakers and who want to look after them properly. Needless to say, I have my own blacklist of venues; I hope that some of the organisers concerned will recognise where they themselves have gone wrong.

(a) The initial letter of invitation should give basic information about the requirements and current level of knowledge of the likely audience and set out the format of the proposed meeting—duration of talk, degree of formality or informality, time allowed for questions, other speakers and their subjects, panel discussion.

(b) The size of the prospective audience should also be given. Speakers are understandably aggrieved if they give up an evening (or indeed any other period of time) and find only a handful of people present. If the attendance is likely to be small and the speaker is told in advance, he or she may well wish to refuse the engagement. My own threshold level is around 20 to 25, but I appreciate that this information is hard to come by and that many organisers are not prepared to commit themselves on this point.

(c) A follow up letter a week or two before the meeting should include directions to the venue. The correct motorway exit is always useful, together with any inside knowledge about the town's inevitable one-way system. For large hospitals, a map showing the position of the lecture theatre is often necessary. Parking problems should be identified and a temporary permit provided if a formal system operates; no lecturer at the end of a hard evening wants to find that his car has been wheel-clamped!

Speakers should be told if a meal is to be provided (before or after the lecture) or whether they are expected to fend for themselves en route. They should also be told if the catering is in any way idiosyncratic—as a confirmed carnivore I find compulsory nut cutlets pretty depressing and I suppose that vegetarians must have the same problems, although perhaps more often.

(d) On the day, the organiser should arrive at the venue before the speaker; it is perhaps surprising how often this does not happen. If the organiser cannot attend, the name of his or her deputy should be sent to the speaker in advance.

(e) Before the start of the meeting, the speaker should be introduced informally to a few selected members of the audience so that he or she starts off feeling welcome and in pleasant company. No speaker should be left standing on their own in a corner, or with only a drug company representative to talk to. Nor should the speaker be saddled with the postgraduate society's most awkward or paranoid member who everyone else is trying to avoid.

(f) if there is no meal attached to the meeting, the speaker should at least be offered a cup of coffee and perhaps a sandwich before or after his or her performance, or both. The distance travelled may have been considerable and perhaps a meal had to be missed to fit in with the time-table.

The speaker should be given the opportunity to visit the toilet before starting. There is nothing worse than getting half way through a planned lecture and feeling that you should have "gone".

(g) When introducing the speaker, the chairperson should be sure about the correct pronunciation of the surname and should also add a first name. It is profoundly discourteous to introduce "Dr Smith" or worse "Dr J Smith", when a single enquiry would allow "Dr John Smith" to be used. A little bit of background biography is also easy for the chairperson to elicit; it is helpful for an audience to be told something of the speaker's credentials.

(h) The speaker will have indicated what is required in the way of visual aids. The organiser should have checked that these are available and in working order, and should know which buttons operate the equipment and lights in the lecture theatre.

(i) The chairperson should have a couple of prepared questions "up his sleeve" in case the discussion period after the formal lecture is slow to get going.

(j) Speakers supported by a major company do not always expect a lecture fee if lecturing is part of their job, but if the engagement is outside normal working hours their goodwill in this respect should not be assumed without due consideration. Doctors from within the NHS who lecture "for love" should certainly receive a proper fee and should be told of the amount in advance. The same criteria apply for the reimbursement of travelling and subsistence expense.

If several doctors appear on the same programme they should all receive the same fee. Speakers naturally tend to congregate together and it is highly embarrassing for one to find that another is receiving a higher (or lower) fee.

(k) If the meeting has been successful the organiser should send a brief "thank you" letter. This simple courtesy particularly applies if no fee has been offered, or if a cheque for a relatively small amount will take three months to arrive from an anonymous NHS or university finance department.

(l) Lastly, the organiser should always remember that the speaker will have had to work hard to prepare the lecture and that he or she may well have had to travel a considerable distance to deliver it, at some personal inconvenience, and with the loss of home comforts. The organiser therefore has an obligation to treat the speaker with courtesy and a duty to provide a sizeable, alert, and inquisitive audience.

Travel to a conference (obtaining funding)

K C B TAN, D J BETTERIDGE

That first major scientific meeting tends never to be forgotten. Because until then, senior, national, and internationally known colleagues are but names on well thumbed papers and reviews. Suddenly there they all are, in the flesh so to speak, either presenting new data or taking part in the discussion of the work of others. Somehow senior figures (at least most of them) seem to be approachable on these occasions and are readily available to give advice and help with scientific matters.

Of course, the occasion can be daunting and sometimes overwhelming if the young research fellow is to present his first paper in front of the leading figures in their subject. Anxious thoughts cross the mind. Have I rehearsed enough? Will I dry up? How does the microphone work? Will I get my slides the wrong way up? Will professor so and so ask difficult questions? etc, etc. It is much better to have sampled the atmosphere of these large meetings—in some specialties there may be over 5000 delegates—before the fateful day of the first paper.

Later in your career the excitement of these meetings pales slightly through familiarity, but they remain a source of intellectual refreshment and ideas. New friendships are made, old ones are renewed, and mutual problems can be discussed. The benefits of attending national, European, and world congresses in your subject are incalculable, and this is especially true for younger people. But raising the money to get to them may seem to be an impossibility. Money can be particularly tight in the research years because available funds only cover payment of the basic salary with no units of medical time. Some of the larger units will have what are commonly called "slush" funds which can be used for funding travel to meetings; such units are relatively few.

So how do you set about raising the necessary money to cover travel and accommodation expenses? Furthermore, the registration fees for meetings seem to be rising exponentially and may well be over £100 a person for a large international meeting.

Funding from the specialist associations

Most specialist associations set aside money, often from major pharmaceutical companies, for the provision of travel grants to junior members. Age limits vary but are usually below 35 years. It is therefore very important to join the appropriate specialist organisation at an early stage. Their funds are, of course, limited and preference is often given to first and second authors of abstracts which have been accepted for presentation at the meeting. Detailed scrutiny of the advance notices for meetings is required as applications for assistance towards travel costs often have to be submitted at the same time as the research abstracts. This can be up to nine months before the meeting. If several abstracts are submitted from a single department some thought as to the order of joint authors can ensure maximum benefit for junior colleagues.

Funding from employers

Travel expenses, subsistence allowances, and registration fees can, in certain circumstances, be obtained from your employer, be it a university, district, or regional health authority, depending on the particular grade of appointment. The overriding principle in negotiating this often tortuous bureaucracy is to plan well in advance. In most cases retrospective claims are not considered. It is not possible to detail here all the regulations concerning study leave and expenses, but enlist the support of your consultant or head of department where appropriate. The postgraduate dean and clinical tutor should point you in the right direction. It is unlikely that junior doctors will receive financial support from health authorities for overseas meetings except in the case of senior registrars presenting their own work. The same restrictions do not apply to university posts, and most universities have funds available for non-tenured staff, although these are strictly limited and often will not cover the full cost of an overseas meeting.

Major grant awarding institutions

It is worth applying to the major grant giving bodies such as the Medical Research Council and the Wellcome Foundation with requests for travel grants, especially if you are already funded by them. Bear in mind, however, that the travel grants awarded by these institutions go mainly to support short visits to other research groups for the exchange of ideas or to learn new techniques. Of course, this important activity could appropriately follow on from a scientific meeting overseas. You must apply well in advance for these awards.

Royal colleges

The royal colleges make travel grants available to members and fellows often in the form of named fellowships. These fellowships provide funds for postgraduate activities and research in prestigious overseas departments for varying lengths of time. They are not primarily designed for attendance at scientific meetings, but a scientific meeting could be an important part of the package of activities.

The Royal Society will consider applications for travel grants from post-doctoral fellows and senior doctors in certain circumstances, so it is worth while obtaining a copy of their regulations.

Pharmaceutical industry

The industry provides considerable funds for travel to and registration at major national and international meetings. This is often done in association with the local organisers of the particular specialist body and the activity is acknowledged in the conference programme. Some pharmaceutical companies also advertise travel grants in the weekly journals, inviting applications which are decided on a competitive basis. In both these instances preference is given to those presenting abstracts which have been accepted for presentation at the meeting.

It is a great advantage for research fellows to have attended one of the major meetings before presenting their own work. But it is much more difficult to obtain funding in this instance unless the particular department where the fellow works has funds available. The pharmaceutical industry may be very useful here. Of course, it helps if the research fellow works in an area in which there is a lot of industry interest. In our view this is a legitimate activity, although some will disagree. Make initial approaches through the relevant local representatives as chances of obtaining funding are often enhanced if the representative is pushing the case. Turn down the offer to discuss this or that product over lunch but tactfully suggest that help towards the travel costs of the next European meeting would be a more worthwhile way to spend the budget.

Make the most of the money raised

Advance programmes for many international scientific meetings provide the facility for booking convenient hotel accommodation beforehand. Furthermore, members of particular speciality associations receive unsolicited details of "package" deals to attend forthcoming major meetings. We have never availed ourselves of these opportunities, believing that good, cheaper alternatives are often possible. This does not apply to national meetings when adequate and cheaper accommodation is to be had in university halls of residence. The traditional "bucket shops" which deal in the "unsold stocks" of airline tickets have been heavily criticised because of financial losses and non-arrival of tickets. But some of these outlets are good and efficient: the difficulty lies in knowing which fall into this category. If you want to deliver your talk to your colleagues at the meeting rather than to other stranded passengers at the airport it is best to use Association of British Travel Agents (ABTA)/International Airline Transport Association (IATA) bonded travel agents whenever possible.

Planning ahead is the most important consideration in obtaining the best deals. Cheaper excursion flights (stay includes a compulsory Saturday night) have to be booked at least two weeks ahead for most European flights and three weeks for those further afield. Consider charter flights/accommodation packages, such as City Breaks, which can be very good value, especially if you share a room with a colleague. Choosing an unpopular flight time (early morning, late night) may enable cheaper tickets to be obtained. For Europe it is worth considering rail travel, and for a small group travelling together driving may prove much cheaper. We know of some colleagues who actually camped out near one European city and travelled in daily for the meeting. For those not so hardy, there are now plenty of available guides which detail cheap and clean basic accommodation in most cities.

Conclusions

It is well worth the challenge to raise money to attend the major meetings in your relevant specialty. An ex-chief known to us refused to give any financial help to his research fellows for travel. His parsimony led to an excellent training in raising money.

Lecture overseas

DAVID LOWE

People's reactions to an invitation to lecture abroad vary. There are those who know they could contribute but see nothing to gain, and those who dream of fame and fortune but don't consider the costs. Some lecturers think, like Nancy Mitford, that "Abroad is unutterably bloody"; others seem to spend only a few weeks a year in the United Kingdom while they arrange their next trip. You will probably be flattered at the invitation, excited by the prospect of travel to foreign parts, faintly nervous at what you might be letting yourself in for, and game enough to suffer at least a little discomfort.

Paperwork

Once you have been invited to lecture abroad and have decided to accept, the first hurdle is to get permission to go. For NHS staff this may simply be a matter of arranging cover with colleagues, but university employees may need the agreement of their dean and head of department as well. Permission to visit may be needed from the host country, and visas should be applied for early. Some consulates take months to process visa applications, and the fact that you simply must attend an international conference of important doctors will cut very little ice. On the application form you should state that you will be delivering a lecture or course of lectures, as this may determine the type of visa that you are given. For example, if there is a fee for the lecture you might not be allowed to accept it if a work visa has not been issued. Most travel insurance policies do not make spearate provision for work abroad rather than tourism, but it is worth checking this. It is important to have medical insurance even if you are the guest of the ministry of health in the host country.

When you are invited somewhere you have never been, many potential difficulties may be avoided if you can speak to someone who has been there. Your hosts may be able to give you names of previous lecturers. In any case try to agree with your hosts what the domestic and procedural arrangements are likely to be, and send them a list of your expectations well before you travel. For example, say that you understand you will be staying in a certain hotel, lecturing for so many hours, having this or that day free, and returning on a particular date. Try to get the address and telephone number of the hotel in which you will be staying so that you can be contacted if an emergency arises at home. Make sure that your hosts know the date and time of your arrival, and remember that days can be gained or lost if you cross the International Date Line.

For lecture courses some hosts arrange broad timings but courteously leave the details to the lecturer; if you are unaware of this you might find that the day of your arrival is spent drawing up a programme. Where possible the course contents and sequence of lectures should be agreed with your hosts and any other visiting lecturers before you go. Planning obviously relies on efficient communications. I once received a letter regretting that my trip had been cancelled four days after my planned departure date.

The way that you lecture will depend to some extent on the audience that you will be addressing. If it is not obvious ask your hosts whether the audience will consist of medical students or postgraduates, generalists or specialists, and whether spouses, non-medical staff, or the press will be invited. Terminology differs among countries. You can look up terms in a textbook in the host country's language. For example, the French and Russians are fond of eponyms, and the names might not be the ones that you are used to. We refer to the Circle of Willis but the French, with more geometrical precision, call it the Polygon.

Audiovisual material

The audiovisual and other material that you take will be determined by your style of lecturing and the information that you wish to convey and also by what facilities will be available at your venue. The equipment can vary from a blackboard without chalk to a three projector split screen *son et lumière* with a choice of independent or simultaneous advance and reverse. If you plan to use slides or overhead projection check that facilities will be available. If you are going to a humid climate remember that glass mounted slides may develop condensation which might boil from the heat of a powerful projector lamp and spoil the acetate.

Lecture notes or handouts prepared before you go will almost always be of better quality than ones photocopied immediately before a lecture, and they do not usually weigh much. When large numbers of notes are needed your hosts may be happy to help with postage or excess baggage charges on the flight, but check with them first.

- Speak slowly
- Show slides slowly
- Limit content of slides
- Say it—and say it again
- Leave time for questions
- Avoid idioms and unusual words
- Avoid lecturing in a foreign language
- Don't tell jokes
- Avoid politics

Foreign currency

You must buy some foreign currency before you go. No matter how well organised a trip is you may find that you have to take a taxi or pay for a meal or drinks because of an unscheduled delay. Some currencies are difficult to obtain so apply to your bank or Thomas Cook as soon as your departure date is confirmed. If you plan to use a credit or charge card to pay for accommodation or meals abroad check that it will be accepted—even large hotels will sometimes not honour them. Hospitality abroad is usually generous, and you might consider taking some small gifts for your hosts, their secretaries, or the car driver.

Travelling out

The saying that to travel hopefully is a better thing than to arrive is rubbish, at least in relation to air travel. It is much better to arrive, and preferably on time. On the day you set off on your trip remember the three most important reasons for frustration and disappointment—delay, delay, and delay. You might use the time to catch up on your reading, assess papers, write book reviews, or draft grant applications. This should confound your detractors who think that lecturing overseas is a holiday.

You must take your slides and other lecture material as hand luggage if possible, so that if your suitcase is delivered to the wrong side of the world you can still give your lecture.

Jet lag can be incapacitating after long journeys. If it is likely to be a problem try to arrange at least one free day at the start of your engagements to recover. Human beings have a "natural" day of 25 hours and jet lag is therefore said to be less when you travel west, but I have never found that this made much difference.

When you arrive at your destination you may wish to be independent and make your own way from the airport to the venue, but in some countries this is unwise and in a few may be dangerous, especially after dark. Try to arrange for someone to meet you.

You can find out what type of climate and temperatures to expect from the broadsheet newspapers, but the intensity of your hotel heating or air conditioning may come as a shock; you can swelter in a Scandinavian winter or shiver in a subtropical summer. The first is easily accommodated by shedding layers of clothing, but consider packing a jumper or cardigan if you go somewhere hot.

Lecturing

There are some points worth considering when you are delivering a lecture to an audience whose language and idiom are not your own:

- Speak slowly. This is more difficult than you might think, especially as you will be enthusiastic about your subject. The expressions on your audience's faces will tell you when you are wasting their time and yours.
- Leave your slides up longer. If the participants are reading and copying from them they may need more time than you expect. You can help by reproducing the written material on the slides as handouts.
- Keep the content of the slides to a minimum, and if necessary use more slides. Use a pointer to identify the areas that you are talking about.
- Follow the pattern of "Say what you are going to say, say it, and

then say what you have said." Be sure to leave time at the end for questions.

- Try to avoid idiomatic phrases, complex sentences, and unusual words. Do not take this to extremes. If you analyse each sentence before you deliver it you will sound awkward and unnatural.
- Avoid lecturing in a foreign language unless you are fluent. It can be disturbing to have the audience giggling at your gaucheries.
- Do not tell jokes or use irony unless you are sure of your audience. At best they may not understand and at worst they will take you seriously.
- Avoid politics. Depending on where you are, this can be embarrassing.

These points are still relevant if you speak British English and your audience speaks American, Canadian, or Indian English, for example, and vice versa: perhaps more so, as you may have an unrealistic sense of well being. In many parts of the world medicine is taught in English, but in European, Far Eastern, and South American countries you may have an interpreter. This is a mixed blessing. Sequential translation disjoints a lecture. Simultaneous translation allows you to lecture relatively normally, but remember that the faster you speak the more rudimentary the translation will be, and there may be mistakes. There may also be a small, tinny voice audible from a nearby set of headphones that stops a second or two after you, which can be very distracting. Give the translator a copy of your lecture the day before. Though you will not deliver it word for word, it will give the interpreter an idea of the contents and of the vocabulary that you are likely to use.

Slides made up in the language of the host country can be used as a courtesy to start or summarise a lecture. Most hospitals have a list of people who will act as translators; consulates can often supply names of professionals whose charges are reasonable.

If you are giving a series of lectures take with you each day from your hotel more material than you think you will need, and be prepared to use less than you had planned. There may be occasions when a lecturer who should speak before you cannot attend, or when the audience wishes to explore a particular point for longer than you had expected. Yoy may also find that you are collected from your hotel with fellow lecturers and have to wait hours before your turn, so take a book.

Coming home

Payment for the work and reimbursement of expenses are usually arranged at the end of the visit. In some places the formalities may take hours. If you are to be paid in soft or local currency rather than sterling or dollars check that you will be able to convert it either at the airport or in your bank at home. You may have to buy goods and export them instead.

Travelling home may be more frustrating than travelling out. Delays seem worse because you are looking forward to seeing family and friends again, the duty free shop may be a disappointment, and you will have spent or changed back all of your local currency and have no hope of buying a cup of tea from the airport café. But you will almost certainly have enjoyed yourself, and when the invitation comes to lecture overseas again next year you will leap at it.

Organise a multicentre trial

C WARLOW

Multicentre and single centre clinical trials share methodological problems which are well known (table I). Multicentre trials do, however, have several distinct advantages. They provide:

- Larger sample size so that the result is more precise, appropriate subgroup analysis is more feasible, and there is a lower risk of an apparently "negative" result when the treatment is, in truth, effective.
- Quicker results before people lose scientific and commercial interest in the treatment, and before it is modified or the theoretical indications for it are changed.
- Wider dissemination of the results and, possibly, more widespread belief in their validity as well.
- Standardised definitions of disease and measurements of outcome among centres and among countries in international trials.
- A wider range of clinical and methodological expertise to solve protocol problems.
- Usually a wider range of patients, facilitating the generalisation of results which can be broadly applied to future patients in other centres and other countries.
- Large "negative" trials which are more likely to be published than small "negative" trials. This is important; otherwise, small "positive" trials, which are more likely to be submitted for publication and probably more likely to be accepted than small "negative" trials, will tend to dominate the scientific literature.
- Less suspicion and rivalry among centres and countries without necessarily suppressing healthy competition.
- Less scientific isolation.
- Better national and international collaboration.

- Facilitation of further multicentre trials of potentially important treatments, provided that the initial trial is not too exhausting.

TABLE I—*Methodological issues common to both single and multicentre trials*

- Randomised or non-randomised treatment comparison
- Blind or open treatment allocation and outcome assessment
- Intention to treat, or on-treatment analysis, or both
- Sample size and duration of follow up
- Subgroup analysis
- Defined entry and exclusion criteria
- Amount of data to collect on randomised and non-randomised but eligible patients
- Defined outcomes
- Widespread applicability of trial results; what to do about non-randomised but eligible patients
- Interim analysis and the role of an independent data monitoring committee
- How intensively to look for adverse effects of treatment
- How intensively to monitor compliance
- Computerisation of data
- Sharing of original data with overview groups looking at similar treatments (meta-analysis)
- Involvement with sponsoring company, if any.

The difficulties of multicentre trials compared with single centre trials mainly concern the coordination of many people in several centres and even countries (table II). There are usually several possible solutions, the best depending on circumstances, geography, number of centres, the budget, and so on. What follows is not meant to be an ossified blue-print but some suggestions— suggestions, moreover, which have not been tested in randomised trials but which, at least, are based on some experience.

TABLE II—*Issues that may present particular difficulties in multicentre trials*

- Leadership
- Writing the protocol
- Finding the centres
- Randomisation
- Patient registration
- Follow up
- Trial coordinator
- Trial office
- Visiting the centres
- Collaborators' meetings
- Quality control
- Cost
- Writing the papers

Leadership

A multicentre trial must have an identifiable leader or principal investigator, who should be able to command the respect of collaborators and have the time and energy to keep the whole enterprise under control. He or she must not lose interest in the dull bit between getting started and getting the results. Running a trial by committee is disastrous. A prestigious chairperson of a steering committee may be a "political" advantage, or even a necessity, but such a person is unlikely to run the trial on a day-to-day basis. Someone must get the funding, gather together centres, run meetings, answer questions, solve problems, visit centres, and set up and supervise the trial office. This person will usually, but not always, be a doctor, presumably whoever wanted to set up the trial in the first place, and someone who is going to be in the same job long enough to see the trial through to the end. A medically qualified principal investigator must try to enter his or her own patients to the trial to maintain credibility, and to experience and share the practical problems with the other collaborators.

Writing the protocol

This is a job for one person, usually the principal investigators, and not a committee. Of course, that person will need comments and advice from all the centres, the trial statistician, and outside experts in the field, and this may all require one or more collaborators' meetings and often several versions of the protocol before everyone is satisfied. Because there is no rule against modifying a protocol if unforeseen problems arise during the trial (provided such modifications are sensible and not dependent on data), there is no reason to delay writing it and getting started while some centres finally make up their minds whether to join in. Indeed, it may be desirable to involve more centres once the trial is underway and some of the teething problems sorted out, although the more centres that are involved from the very start the better. It does not always hold, however, that centres involved in writing the protocol are more likely to stick to it than centres joining later and having to accept it. In international trials the protocol may have to be translated into several languages which can be surprisingly expensive. Fortunately, if it is written in English, translation is now hardly necessary, at least not in western Europe, which is a huge advantage to us in Great Britain and a great credit to our medical colleagues on the continent.

Finding the centres

Having accepted that a multicentre rather than a single-centre trial is scientifically necessary to solve a particular treatment problem, friends and colleagues from a few centres usually get together to discuss a protocol. From there, other friends and colleagues are brought in from centre to centre, and from country to country until enough centres are found to satisfy the sample size requirements in a reasonable period of time. After about three years recruitment gets tedious and may fall off, but follow up is usually less time consuming and may need to continue much longer, depending on the treatment. Key people in a country are often very successful in recruiting their own compatriots, far more so than an outsider. Advertising in medical journals and through specialist organisations can also help. Pharmaceutical companies may, through their national and international networks, approach numerous potential collaborators simultaneously.

However the centres are found, they must be seriously interested and reasonably competent in the field, but not necessarily specialists. In any event specialists may already be involved in their own competing studies; relative non-specialists in district general hospitals or general practice may be extremely keen to collaborate—and make very effective collaborators. Usually they have more patients than teaching hospitals, they may have no other way to take part in medical research, and to be involved with specialists in the field who are organising the trial is often educative. But whoever the collaborators are, they are all equal when it comes to recruiting patients and it is *their* trial, not the principal investigator's whose role is organisational and catalytic: there should be no "star billing".

Randomisation

This must be centralised and is best done by telephone, or perhaps by a computer link, to some central point which may be the trial office or, if 24 hour cover is required, a hospital ward or switchboard. This is the only way for the trial organisers to have an immediate binding record of who has been randomised, when, and from which centre. Sealed envelopes or locally held randomisation lists are simply not good enough.

Patient registration

If large numbers are required and the budget is limited patient registration must be simple, practical, and quick. Collaborators should have to do little more than what is normally required in routine clinical practice. Patients must be identified (name, sex, date of birth), data on a few important prognostic variables collected, and possible prespecified subgroups identified. It is often feasible to collect all or some of these data on the telephone before treatment allocation is made, so obviating the need to complete, post, check, code and punch data entry forms. It also means that the treatment allocation is not made unless and until the entry data are recorded centrally. Another advantage is that data recorded *before* randomisation are unbiased with respect to any knowledge of treatment allocation. Computer networks which do the same thing are another possibility, but more expensive. Superfluous data must not be collected and nor should "add on" studies be allowed without adequate human and financial resources. Indeed, all the collaborators must have a very clear idea of the aim of the trial and concentrate on that. Nevertheless, it may be possible for a few particularly interested collaborators to collect more data than the others, but this should be optional and certainly not to the detriment of patient recruitment or answering the basic trial question.

Follow up

This must also be simple and require little more than would be done in routine clinical practice. Obviously, the outcome must be recorded and measured but this may not require frequent follow up, and sometimes it can be obtained from routinely collected data (such as death certificates, cancer registries, etc.), thus disposing with the need for follow up at all. Some follow up might be more simply, and even more accurately, obtained by telephoning the patient rather than by contacting the patient's doctor. Overelaborate recording of and testing compliance should be avoided as should unnecessary blood tests. Too frequent and too detailed follow up may add very little to the statistical power and may kill recruitment in a multicentre trial once trial contributors realise what they have let themselves in for. Written forms should be no longer than one side of A4 paper; if they are, they probably will not be completed fully or reliably. In any event trials should not interfere with routine clinical practice.

Trial coordinator

This is the key person even if the trial is not large enough to merit a full time appointment. The job is administrative, not medical. She, for it is seldom he, stands at the centre of the trial and must be committed, energetic, sensible, well organised, have some knowledge of computing, and be able to work flexible hours. To collect the data, organise them, and transmit them to the statistician she must be meticulous and even obsessional but she must also be good with people so that she can run the trial office and maintain harmonious relationships with the distant collaborators. She must be adroit at dealing with the awkward (and some doctors can be remarkably awkward) and flexible and energetic enough so that she can hop on and off trains and planes and put up with a certain amount of discomfort as she travels from centre to centre extracting data from forgetful collaborators, encouraging them to randomise more patients, and generally nurturing esprit-de-corps, while still retaining a sense of humour.

Trial office

The trial office, organised and supervised by the trial coordinator, has the task of collecting, checking, and entering the data from the distant centres and requesting more information if there are inconsistencies or omissions. The office must supply the collaborators with all the necessary documentation (entry and follow up forms, freepost envelopes, sticky labels, etc.) and possibly even the trial medication, dispatch regular newsletters and listings on missing data and listings of when patients are due for their next follow up, and answer questions from the many centres. The office must be available, friendly, helpful, knowledgeable, reliable and efficient, perhaps in more than one language for international trials; although doctors may speak excellent English, the same does not necessarily apply to their hospital telephonists. The collaborators must see the office as a "black box" into which data go in and out of which information comes. Any strife, inefficiency, or chaos should remain hidden. Such an office needs to be close to the principal investigator and, if possible, to the statistician, although with the availability of modern high speed computer links this may not be so important now. The office requires secretarial and clerical staff, a telephone and answering machine independent of a busy hospital or university switchboard, a Fax machine, a photocopier, several microcomputers, printers, filing cabinets and adequate storage space. It must have enough resources to do its job properly and take as much as possible of the burden of the trial organisation from the collaborators. The resources required will gradually increase through the recruitment period, after which they will stabilise, but probably not decline.

Visiting the centres

This is time consuming and expensive but must be done, often regularly, for the following reasons: (i) to discuss any local problems arising from understanding and implementing the protocol; (ii) encourage recruitment to the trial and solve problems relating to this; collect outstanding data, although with advance warning these usually appear in the trial office shortly before the visit; (iii) discover neighbouring centres interested in joining the trial; (iv) reinforce the role of each centre without which the trial would fail; and (v) to keep everyone informed of what is going on in the trial as a whole. The meeting must be arranged well in advance because it is important to get *all* the local collaborators around a table. But the visit need not last long, perhaps an hour or so. Remember, the local collaborators are busy and the trial is unlikely to be their major preoccupation or priority. Who does the visits depends on the circumstances; the trial coordinator is usually the best person to collect data and the principal investigator best at sorting out scientific and medical problems, but a regional coordinator can be helpful if the centres are widely dispersed. Whoever it is must not waste time; several centres can often be visited in a day and work can be done on trains. Trains with sleeping compartments allow an early start to the day to be made. Avoid visits during the summer when collaborators are on holiday and the trains are full of additional passengers and avoid the depths of winter when snow and fog dislocate transport. Don't carry too much with you but take enough to read in case you get delayed;

take train and 'plane timetables and be prepared to change your plans; sort out how to get money quickly in foreign countries; and make sure the trial office and your family know your whereabouts.

Collaborators' meetings

These are needed to write, and if necessary, rewrite the protocol; to discuss disease definitions, measurements of outcome, and documentation; to discuss any interim results; to encourage treatment; to plan new trials; and to encourage a group identity and common purpose. They are, however, time consuming to attend, extremely time consuming to organise, and expensive. They should therefore be frequent enough to fulfil their purpose, but not so frequent as to be prohibitively expensive. It may be sensible—or even essential—to organise regional or national collaborators' meetings if there are a large number of widely dispersed centres. It may also be possible to link trial meetings to others that collaborators are likely to be going to anyway, such as national specialist societies, international meetings, etc. Furthermore, it may be scientifically attractive (and indeed commercially attractive if registration fees and sponsorship are forthcoming) to organise a symposium or educational meeting alongside the trial meeting.

Quality control

In a single centre trial it is important that the trial treatment is properly described, well delivered, and any complications fairly assessed. This is even more important in multicentre trials where there are certain to be differences among centres, both real and due to chance. Even trial drug treatment may differ because of different storage conditions or possibly circumstances of delivering it to the patients. But of more concern is variation among centres in non-drug treatments being evaluated, such as surgery, speech therapy, psychotherapy, etc. Obviously all the centres must agree to standardise more or less such treatments so that about the same amount is given, for about the same time, and that it is reasonably uniform. Such non-drug treatments, however, will never be *exactly* the same in all centres and it is counter-productive to insist that they are; as long as they are roughly similar no problems will arise and the trial result will be applicable to other centres giving roughly, but never *exactly*, the same treatment. Monitoring uniformity of treatment is difficult but at least it helps to monitor any immediate complications, such as postoperative morbidity, and to have regular meetings of the collaborators. If a centre is performing badly (inadequate treatment, excessive complications, not enough patients to ensure competence, etc.) then it should stop randomising patients, but not, of course, stop following up those already randomised. Clinically sensible co-interventions, such as drug regimens administered during a trial of a surgical procedure, do not have to be exactly the same in each centre because randomisation (statified by centre if necessary) will ensure that they are used in the same proportion of "treated" and "control" patients across the trial participants. In a multicentre trial there may actually be more strenuous efforts made than in a single centre trial to ensure that the treatment (both trial and co-intervention) is properly delivered and discussed, so that generalising the results may actually be more appropriate; in a single centre trial the treatment programme may be less likely to be submitted to peer review, criticism, and audit.

Cost

Multicentre trials are expensive but they need not be prohibitively so provided the collaborators are reasonable and do not attempt to re-equip their entire department and undertake major non-trial projects at the expense of a sponsoring pharmaceutical company. Indeed, from the point of view of unit cost per patient randomised, or per patient year of follow up, multicentre trials should be cheaper than single centre trials as they gain from economies of scale. But, of course, the trial office and collaborators' meetings must be properly funded and the collaborators themselves reimbursed for any extra work (which is very little in a well designed trial) over and above routine clinical practice. There are various ways of doing this: a lump sum for every patient randomised; a sum for every completed data form received by the trial office; a formula based on the number of patients randomised to support a research nurse, etc. Whatever is done, the collaborators should be paid only for extra work done, and not work that they say they will do. In many trials, however, it is very difficult to obtain proper funding. This applies particularly to treatments from which no profits are to be made—for example, non-patented drugs, surgery, physiotherapy, etc.—so that it is totally inappropriate for trial funding to be left entirely to the pharmaceutical industry. Although a sponsoring company must not be involved in either data analysis or publication, it can be extremely helpful in collecting baseline (but *not* outcome) data, maintaining trial discipline, and encouraging recruitment through its own networks of medical representatives and researchers. Whatever the cost of a trial, it should be compared with the incidence, prevalence, and cost of the disease being treated and, perhaps, against the cost of non-medical endeavours such as low altitude military aircraft training or unemployment benefit. By any such comparisons, multicentre trials are usually extremely inexpensive and may lead to the rejection of expensive but ineffective treatments—for example, extracranial to intracranial bypass surgery for the prevention of stroke—and not always to the introduction of more expensive health care.

Writing the papers

Like the protocol, this is a job for the principal investigator, not a committee. Naturally, it will be necessary to have many discussions with the trial statistician and trial coordinator and comments and advice from all the collaborators as numerous drafts are produced. It is crucial, however, that in the end all the results are published under the name of all the collaborators: without them there would have been no trial at all and they did the work. Although currently unfashionable in some quarters, the whole philosophy underlying multicentre trials is that group effort takes precedence over individual effort: only by acting as a group can the individuals get answers to therapeutic questions which affect their own individual patients. Of course, any centre can publish its *own* results but there must be no "star billing" for authors when the results of the whole trial are presented.

Conclusions

Before starting a multicentre trial the following questions must be answered affirmatively: Is the therapeutic question really important, preferably even a burning issue? Are you sure there is no better way of answering it? Can you get enough centres together? Are you likely to get the resources? Have you got the time? Do you *really* want to do it? If so, then go ahead, but first visit one or two successful multicentre trial organisations which will give you far more idea of the problems and pleasures than I have been able to within the context of this article. Remember, only fools fail to learn from others' mistakes. And once you get started, always keep thinking about how the trial can be done more efficiently and effectively, less expensively, more quickly with a greater recruitment rate and with less extra work being done by the collaborators. At the same time, remember that esprit-de-corps is what counts more than anything else: look after it.

Set up a coronary rehabilitation programme

H J N BETHELL

Supervised rehabilitation for patients who are recovering from coronary illness or coronary surgery could and should be provided by every district general hospital. It would not be expensive to do so, but requires the hospital cardiologists and physicians to initiate, encourage, and nurture the programmes.

Why do it?

Coronary rehabilitation, which is popular in many Western countries, is not widely available in the United Kingdom. Although most cardiologists and general physicians support the concept, few are sufficiently interested to initiate rehabilitation programmes. Such treatment is, however, of great value in helping patients who have had an infarct or bypass graft to cope with the problems that face them. They are usually physically unfit, partly because few will have been taking regular exercise and partly because the period of rest necessary after the acute event produces further deconditioning. Patients are often depressed by the threat to their future and security and nearly always anxious about the chance of a recurrence. They suffer various symptoms such as "missed beats" and niggling left sided chest pains, which further undermine their battered self confidence. Angina or breathlessness may appreciably impair their exercise tolerance. A return to work provides an immense hurdle for many manual workers for whom a degree of physical fitness may be vital to the retention of their jobs.

Despite these difficulties most patients recover from their infarction or cardiac surgery and return to a reasonable level of functioning, though this is usually well below their optimal performance.

The rate of return to work of patients who have had coronary artery bypass is disturbingly low, and a substantial minority of patients who have had an infarct do poorly because of continued depression or anxiety. (Half of those who are not back at work six months after the attack are suffering from cardiac neurosis rather than physical disability.) A well organised rehabilitation programme can tackle all these problems and also provide a setting for other secondary preventive measures such as giving up smoking, changing the diet, and so on.

What should be done?

The core of coronary rehabilitation is physical training to ease the patient from inactivity back to full activity as quickly and safely as possible. Getting the patient mobilised early on in hospital and encouraging an optimistic attitude towards future physical capacity sets the scene, and this can be backed up by videos showing patients taking part in rehabilitation and by visits from former patients who have had this treatment.

Most patients are ready to start graduated exercise within three or four weeks of infarction and within five or six weeks of coronary artery surgery. The initial assessment includes taking a history, examining the patient, and taking a resting electrocardiogram. Patients who have increasing angina, heart failure, or uncontrolled arrhythmias should be sent back to their physician for further treatment. An exercise test should be carried out with electrocardiographic monitoring using either a treadmill or a bicycle ergometer. The treadmill provides an exercise to which the patient is accustomed, but it is expensive, noisy, and space consuming and some patients find it difficult to balance on one. The bicycle is cheap and easy to operate and allows blood pressure to be measured accurately during the test but requires the patient to keep a constant pedalling rate. It is usual to take the patient up to 85% of his or her predicted maximum heart rate or to level 5 or 6 on the Borg scale for those who are taking β blockers, unless stopped by angina, excessive breathlessness, falling blood pressure, or complex arrhythmias. (The Borg scale is a scoring system for perceived exertion, which runs from 0.5 (very, very light) to 10 (very, very heavy) and which has been shown to have a good correlation with heart rate response to exercise.) Problems arising during the test may indicate the need for further treatment before

123

starting exercise. The test measures the present fitness level from which the exercise prescription can be devised and against which future performance can be compared.

The exercises used should be dynamic or "aerobic"—that is, entailing much movement without emphasising power. Such exercise raises the heart rate and systolic blood pressure and produces breathlessness. Isometric exercise involves strength rather than movement, raises both systolic and diastolic pressure without great effect on the heart rate, and has much less effect on aerobic fitness which is so desirable for the coronary patient. The most popular regimen in Britain is circuit training using various exercises such as stationary cycling, stepping up and down, jogging on a mini-trampoline, and a mix of arm and leg exercises with light dumb bells. This is easy to supervise in a small area and needs little equipment. The variety provided by a circuit is less boring than single exercise sessions, reduces the risk of musculoskeletal injuries, and prepares the patient for many different activities at work and leisure. Some centres do rely on a single exercise such as cycling or jogging and find it satisfactory. A warm up routine with non-competitive games may enjoyably round up the session.

The training sessions should ideally be held three or four times a week (but twice a week will suffice), last 20 to 30 minutes, and increase the heart rate to between 70% and 85% of the patient's predicted maximum (85% of the predicted maximum heart rate is roughly 195 minus the age) or to a lower heart rate if indicated by the exercise test—in patients taking β blockers or with angina. This regimen has been shown to be optimal for producing a good increase in fitness; more frequent, prolonged, or intensive exertion gives little further benefit but carries an increased risk of musculoskeletal injuries or undesirable cardiac arrhythmias. The patient starts with a very light circuit and this is increased gradually in number and speed of repetitions in response to the heart rate reached at the previous session. It is helpful to encourage the spouse to join in the training programme, giving him or her an insight into the patient's exercise capacity, thus reducing "mollycoddling" at home and encouraging compliance. Within two or three weeks home exercise should be started since wholly supervised sessions encourage dependence and a high dropout rate once the course is over. The home sessions can include a circuit similar to the supervised ones using 3 kg dumb bells for arm and leg movements, jogging on the spot, and stepping up and down two steps.

Coronary rehabilitation		
Why?	*When?*	*What?*
Patients	Start:	Assessment
• unfit	• 3–4 weeks after	Aerobic exercise (usually
• anxious	myocardial infarction	circuit training)
• functioning below	• 5–6 weeks after	
optimal level	coronary artery surgery	Aim to increase heart rate
• angina/breathlessness		to 75–85% of predicted
	Sessions 20–30 minutes	maximum
Secondary prevention	2–4 times a week for 6–	
	12 weeks	Involve spouse
	Continue exercise at home	

Many patients have or can borrow a static bicycle or rowing machine which may be incorporated into the circuit. The heart rate before and after exercise and the time taken to complete the exercise are recorded so that logical progression can be worked out. A daily brisk walk over a measured distance of one to two miles recording the same observations is a useful extra and in fitter patients can be increased to a jog within a few weeks.

The length of the course must depend on local resources and the number of patients presenting for treatment. Six to 12 weeks is usual—it is long enough to increase fitness moderately and to start the patient on the road to continued unsupervised exercise as part of the way of life. This duration must be flexible to allow for those with little heart damage who progress very quickly and for those with cardiac or psychological problems who need much more careful nurturing through the programme. A final exercise test to measure the fitness level attained can be followed by the long term exercise prescription.

Who should do it and where?

There is no reason why every district general hospital in Britain should not provide this facility for patients after an infarct or coronary artery surgery. A cardiologist or general physician who is interested in cardiac rehabilitation would be the most suitable person to organise it. In most hospitals, however, there is no one who is sufficiently motivated to do it, which explains why there are so few programmes. In several hospitals a nurse or physiotherapist has initiated a rehabilitation course which has then been supported with more or less enthusiasm by the doctors. Each district general hospital serves a population of several hundred general practitioners, and where it is not possible to find a member of the hospital staff to do it it should be easy to find a local general practitioner to take it on. The general practitioner would usually need to be recruited by the hospital, though some might initiate programmes themselves.

There is no course of instruction in Britain for would-be cardiac rehabilitators. Some necessary areas of knowledge include coronary heart disease, exercise physiology, exercise testing, the special problems of exercise in coronary patients, and resuscitation. Most people who are interested in this subject will have experience in some of these disciplines, but most will need to extend their education by visiting existing programmes, cardiac departments, and exercise laboratories and by reading (a suggested reading list is given at the end of this paper).

The physiotherapy department is the obvious place for holding courses in hospital. Outside hospital community sports centres provide the ideal site. Not only do they have more space than most hospitals but they also have much of the appropriate equipment for circuit training, often including bicycle ergometers, and have staff well experienced in using it. An added advantage of exercising at sports centres is that it encourages a return to normal. The patient going to the sports centre is having fun rather than treatment, and this should encourage compliance and in the long term lead to a habit of regular exercise.

What does it cost?

The minimum equipment includes a defibrillator and oscilloscope (c £3000), and one or two bicycle ergometers (c £400 each), and a few exercise accessories such as dumb bells, barbels, two step climbs, and minitrampolines (not more than £300). For hospital courses only the exercise equipment will need to be bought. The defibrillator and oscilloscope provides the main financial hurdle for the programme outside hospital, but these can often be borrowed from the hospital. Public interest in community coronary rehabilitation makes it easy to raise charitable funds for equipment.

The Basingstoke District Hospital course employs two hospital practitioner sessions (£3700 a year), a sports officer for three hours a week (£707 a year), and a physiotherapist for three hours a week (£877 a year), giving a grand total of £5284 a year. About 100 patients are treated each year, making the cost per rehabilitated patient £53, less than the cost of half a day in hospital.

What else should be done?

Patients who are recovering from heart attacks or heart surgery have needs beyond simply regaining physical fitness. They are usually anxious to take all possible steps to reduce the chance of further coronary problems, and they gratefully embrace all approaches which may help. Most will have given up smoking in the coronary care unit, but those who have not will need help. Dietary advice to help reduce weight and where appropriate to reduce blood fat concentrations should be provided. Teaching patients about the nature of coronary heart disease, its risk factors, symptoms, and logical management helps them to understand their condition and to work for their own good health. The group therapy effect of the rehabilitation sessions, which provide the opportunity for patients to meet and discuss mutual difficulties, makes it easier for them to cope with minor problems. Severe tension, anxiety, and depression, which may not readily be admitted, need to be recognised and will often require professional treatment. Ideally, counselling and management of stress, and later on help with the return to work, should be available. Finally, once the patients have finished the supervised rehabilitation it should be easy for them to continue to exercise, preferably as a group. Organising a self help club of graduates of the course is the best way of catering for their need for exercise, social support, and recreation.

References

Andersen E L, Shephard R J, Denolin H, Varnauskas E, Masironi F. *Fundamentals of exercise testing.* Geneva: World Health Organisation, 1971.

Astrand P-O, Rodahl K. *Textbook of work physiology.* New York: McGraw-Hill, 1976.

Clausen J C. Effect of physical training on cardiovascular adjustments to exercise in man. *Physiol Rev* 1977; **57**: 779–815.

Joint Working Party of the Royal College of Physicians of London and the British Cardiac Society. Cardiac rehabilitation 1975. *J R Coll Physicians Lond* 1975; **9**: 281–346.

Scientific Council on Rehabilitation of Cardiac Patients. *Myocardial infarction. How to prevent. How to rehabilitate.* International Society and Federation of Cardiology, 1983.

Shephard R J. *Ischaemic heart disease and exercise.* London: Croom Helm, 1981.

Wenger N K, Hellerstein H K, eds. *Rehabilitation of the coronary patient.* New York: Wiley, 1978.

Start a DNA diagnostic service

K F KELLY, N E HAITES, A W JOHNSTON

In 1985 the Scottish Home and Health Department allocated funds under the New Developments in Health Care Programme to establish a national molecular genetics diagnostic service with laboratories in four university cities: Glasgow, Edinburgh, Dundee, and Aberdeen. Each centre would be responsible for the diagnosis of certain diseases for the whole of Scotland, and centres would cooperate by collecting blood and extracting DNA and dispatching it to one of the laboratories for analysis. Each centre would be responsible for counselling and investigating patients in their areas. The laboratories would thus act as a consortium with considerable contact and cooperation, sharing work, and avoiding expensive duplication of services.

The disorders to be diagnosed were allocated in a way that reflected a research or clinical interest that already existed—for example, X linked muscular dystrophies to Glasgow. Other diseases allocated were cystic fibrosis and Huntington's disease to Edinburgh, dystrophia myotonica to Aberdeen, and adult polycystic kidney disease to Dundee.

Our laboratory is associated with the Cytogenetics Service, which covers the whole Grampian region. In this brief description of the first two years our service has operated we include practical advice on setting up a molecular genetics service.

Our primary aim was to establish the necessary laboratory procedures and to acquire the probes needed to fulfil our commitment. About 100 blood samples from patients affected by various diseases, notably Huntington's disease and muscular dystrophies, had already been stored by the clinical geneticists before the laboratory was established. We were therefore quickly able to provide DNA

TABLE I—*Sample intake for 1986 and 1987 (numbers given) in Aberdeen, showing some of the principal disorders and diagnostic centres in Scotland*

Disorder	1986	1987	Analysis possible	Centre
Huntington's disease	93	54	Yes	Edinburgh
Duchenne muscular dystrophy	33	18	Yes	Glasgow
Becker muscular dystrophy	0	9	Yes	Glasgow
Dystrophia myotonica	12	63	Yes	Aberdeen
Cystic fibrosis	5	19	Yes	Edinburgh
Adult polycystic kidney disease	0	14	Yes	Dundee
Fragile X	6	18	Not yet	Aberdeen
Hypercholesterolaemia	0	16	Yes	Aberdeen
Others	65	165		

Note: The 1987 figures represent the intake up to December 1987.

from families with muscular dystrophy for analysis in Glasgow. Soon after work started and probes became available clinicians began sending in blood samples from families. Table I shows some of the disorders for which we have been asked to prepare DNA, with the numbers of samples for 1986 and 1987. Several local families were known to have dystrophia myotonica, so this disease was used to test the development of our laboratory techniques. The probes that we now have which proved useful in the diagnosis of dystrophia myotonica were donated by research laboratories in the United Kingdom and The Netherlands.

Laboratory service

Staffing—A postdoctoral scientist with five years' experience in molecular biology and a graduate technician are in charge of our laboratory. Another technician will soon be required. We believe that at least two scientists are needed to provide an effective core group.

Accommodation—The molecular genetics service was allocated a small office and a laboratory (36.5 m²) which is adequate for preparing DNA, restriction analysis, and gel electrophoresis. Additional laboratory space is required for the microbiological and isotope work necessary for preparing probes.

Equipment—In the first year basic equipment was obtained for our exclusive use. In addition to bench top centrifuges a versatile centrifuge such as the Sorvall RC5C is invaluable for preparing

TABLE II—*Basic equipment required in a molecular genetics laboratory*

1	Bacteriology facilities for probe propagation and preparation—for example, an incubator where cultures can be grown
2	Preparative, benchtop, and microcentrifuges are necessary for plasmid isolation, DNA preparation, and handling the very small volumes of solution in restriction digestion procedures
3	Gilson type micropipettes are essential for restriction digestion, probe labelling, and many other purposes
4	Variable temperature waterbaths are required for restriction digestions and hybridisation procedures
5	Electrophoresis equipment should include at least two powerpacks with gel beds of various sizes. Many types are available (BRL, Pharmacia LKB)
6	Darkroom facilities should include an ultraviolet light source and camera to record the appearance of gels, and x-ray cassettes are necessary for autoradiography
7	Fridges and freezers are required to store samples and chemicals such as DNA and restriction enzymes, a minimum requirement would be a $-20°C$ freezer and a $-70°C$ freezer

Note: This list is not comprehensive, but these items would be required for the exclusive use of a diagnostic service. Absolute numbers depend on finance available to equip a new laboratory. Consideration should be given to laboratory space, which is required for microbiology (probe preparation) and isotope handling and disposal. Separate rooms are ideal.

probes and genomic DNA. For restriction analysis it is necessary to have microcentrifuges, a set of micropipettes, and variable temperature waterbaths for digests and hybridisations. Two powerpacks are needed with three or four gel tanks, one being of the "baby gel" type for probe sequence isolation. Such basic equipment might cost about £15 000. Automated DNA extraction should allow a much larger sample load to be handled at an additional cost of about £30 000. Table II lists the basic equipment required in a molecular genetic diagnostic laboratory. The annual running costs, based on our figures and covering isotope, enzymes, hybridisation membranes, and chemicals, would be about £6000–7000.

Methods—Practical experience has to be acquired before reliable techniques can be established. We found valuable the descriptions in the publications cited in table III, where the necessary details for all the techniques are given.

DNA probes—To obtain many probes it is necessary to write directly to the originator, but requests for diagnostic use are rarely refused. Some probes may be obtained from the American Type Culture Collection, Rockville, Maryland, for about $50 each. The

TABLE III—*Publications and basic techniques which are practically useful*

Useful publications:
Maniatis T, *et al. Molecular cloning, a laboratory manual.* Cold Spring Harbor, New
York: Cold Spring Harbor Laboratory Press, 1982
The Practical Approach Series. IRL Press, Oxford (especially Davies K E. *Human
genetic diseases,* 1986)

DNA extraction methods:
Kunkel L, *et al.* Whole blood. *Proc Natl Acad Sci.* USA 1977; **74**: 1254
Old J. Chorion villus, In: Davies K E, ed. *Human genetic diseases.* Oxford: IRL
Press, 1986

Restriction enzyme digestion of genomic DNA:
4–5 μg of DNA with 20–25 units of enzyme in a total volume of 30 μl.
Incubate for 5 hours or overnight. Follow manufacturers' instructions for buffer
compositions

Labelling of DNA:
Oligolabelling is efficient and simple. Kits are available commercially or nucleotide
mixes can be prepared in the laboratory: both work well. Klenow enzyme is
required. Feinberg A P, Vogelstein B. *Anal Biochem* 1984; **137**: 266

Hybridisation membranes:
We have found Hybond-N and GeneScreen Plus/Amersham and NEN) satisfactory. In the prehybridisation and hybridisation solutions BSA can be replaced
with powdered milk to give good blocking

Autoradiography:
We use commercially available cassettes with two intensifying screens and standard
x-ray film. Exposure is for 2–3 days at -70°C

name of a laboratory staff member must be sent to the ATCC
before they will accept an order from their catalogue. Many probes
are obtained as plasmids in bacterial hosts so permanent stocks
have to be established, genotypes tested, and amplified probe
DNA made. Good microbial practices are essential at this early
stage so that valuable probe stocks are not contaminated.

Preparation of genomic DNA—Preparing genomic DNA from
blood and tissue by the method of Kunkel *et al* (table III) has
proved perfectly satisfactory. For cleaning up the DNA after pro-
teinase digestion we use redistilled phenol, available commercially,
rather than impure grades which may affect restriction enzyme
activity. Digestion of genomic DNA carried out overnight using
four to fivefold excess of enzyme (1 μg DNA to 4–5 units of
enzyme) normally works well. It is important that digestion goes to
completion to avoid misdiagnoses owing to the presence of the
products of partial digestion. DNA can be stored in TE buffer at
4°, -20°, or -70°C in 1.5 ml Eppendorf type tubes.

Hybridisation methods—In a laboratory starting up from scratch hybridisation may cause the most problems. We found that the main difficulties arose in labelling the probe DNA and in achieving good hybridisation signals free from background contamination. Except in one or two special cases, such as minisatellite repeat probes, the best method for labelling probes is the random oligonucleotide priming technique of Feinberg and Vogelstein (table III). This requires that isolated probe sequence is prepared on a low melting point agarose gel, but very small amounts of probe DNA can be labelled efficiently by this method. Of the many methods and types of filter material available, we have used and obtained good results with the nylon membranes Hybond and GeneScreen Plus. Before experimenting with other hybridisation methods it is wise in the first instance simply to follow the manufacturer's instructions. Although the methods may not be the most rapid, they are well tested and reliable. Southern blotting itself rarely poses problems, but inefficient prehybridisation (the process which blocks membrane sites, thus reducing non-specific probe binding) may do. Care is required here and in the preparation of pure probe to ensure that no non-probe sequences are labelled. We are currently testing a blot processor system for diagnostic use. In this system special bags are provided that have stoppered ports through which solutions can be added and removed. By attaching a pump, filters can be washed rapidly and efficiently and the special holding apparatus cuts down the operator's exposure to radioactivity.

Practical problems—Although the laboratory staff were experienced in the techniques of restriction digestion, Southern blotting, and hybridisation, some problems were encountered, particularly in the hybridisation steps, which caused considerable frustration. Usually there was no clear reason why an analysis would fail, but about nine months were spent testing out membrane samples and prehybridisation, hybridisation, and labelling conditions until methods suitable and *robust* enough for use were developed. Problems in the setting up stages in new laboratories are not uncommon and should be expected.

Procedure time—We now expect to be able to produce a result—that is, identify a marker for the disease if it is present—within 10–12 days of receiving a blood sample (assuming that no technical problems occur and that we have the correct probes). Analyses are not undertaken until samples are available from appropriate family members.

Clinical considerations

While the clinical geneticists were delighted to make use of the consortium to improve the service to the patients attending the genetic clinic in Aberdeen, several hurdles needed to be overcome to make efficient use of its facilities. One was the need to have other clinicians educated to understand how current molecular biology techniques could be used to keep this information updated—no mean feat in a discipline where rapid progress is being made.

Another is the need to carry out extended family studies to obtain the maximum information from DNA analysis. Many probes do not detect the exact location of the affected gene but detect sequences that are sufficiently close on the chromosome that they have a high probability of being inherited with that gene (they are therefore known as linked probes). Family studies are essential so that the marker patterns (restriction fragment length polymorphisms or RFLPs) from both affected and unaffected members can be identified—that is, the family made informative. Since in this form of analysis it is rarely possible to do individual tests, we have sought cooperation from physicians, paediatricians, ophthalmologists, general practitioners, and others. It has also been necessary to contact doctors in other parts of Scotland to speak to a family and where possible obtain blood. Blood samples to make a local family informative have arrived from as far afield as the United States.

Difficulties may also arise in explaining to the referred members of the family the reason why other members have to be involved and, to them, why they, who are often unaffected or spouses, need to give blood. Remarkably, most members of families seem to be delighted to be involved for the good of a few. But because of fear of the unknown or a family disagreement some have refused. This type of clinical work is extremely time consuming. For each family group several consultations are required to ensure that all members of the family are fully informed and have understood the nature of the test, the results it may produce, and especially the limitations of the analysis. Once results are available for a family further counselling is required to discuss the implications for each member.

For the dystrophia myotonica families studied so far our results have confirmed the unaffected state of many individuals at high risk of carrying the abnormal gene and established the affected state of some whose signs were so slight—early cataracts and slight electromyographic changes—that the diagnosis could easily be overlooked. Several family groups have now been made informative for prenatal diagnosis. This is of particular relevance to women who, even when mildly affected, may have children with a severe form of this disease which may result in neonatal death. Figure 1 shows a pedigree from a family informative with the linked probe APOC2 in a two polymorphism analysis.

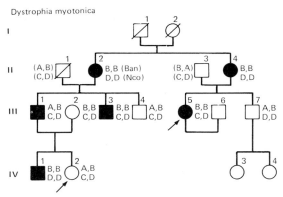

Fig 1—*Pedigree of a family with dystrophia myotonica. The condition is segregating with haplotype B, D, and the clinically normal propositus IV-2 has a 96% chance of having inherited the normal gene. Propositus III-5 could be informative for prenatal diagnosis.*

In another autosomal dominant condition, familial hypercholesterolaemia, the diagnosis can be made in children before abnormal lipid profiles are noted. This allows dietary control before incorrect eating habits are acquired. Figure 2 shows a pedigree where this condition was identified in a young child by means of restriction fragment length polymorphism analysis using part of the low density lipoprotein receptor gene as a probe. In the past year results from other members of the consortium have contributed to the management of families in the Aberdeen area with individuals suffering from inherited diseases such as Duchenne muscular dystrophy, cystic fibrosis, and adult polycystic kidney disease.

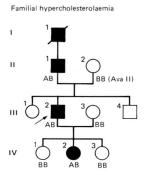

Familial hypercholesterolaemia

Fig 2—*Pedigree of a family with familial hypercholesterolaemia. The condition is segregating with the paternal A allele, and thus IV-2 has a high risk of being affected.*

Discussion

We think it is essential that in addition to laboratory facilities for diagnosing genetic disorders there is also sufficient clinical support. When prenatal diagnosis is being considered the whole family should be investigated in the genetic clinic before another pregnancy is considered to ensure that an informative polymorphism is available for that family. Similarly, if the disease cannot be investigated by the laboratory another unit must be approached or the necessary probes obtained and prepared, otherwise there may be undue haste or delay, or both. In identifying families who require the service of a molecular genetics laboratory the cooperation of many people, particularly the family doctors, is of great importance. The ability to provide advice rapidly to anxious families depends on the closest liaison between the DNA laboratory and the clinical geneticist. This is greatly facilitated by the medical and laboratory staff being located close together, so that the best possible approach to diagnosis for a particular family can be easily discussed.

The numbers of families identified and tested for a particular disorder in a region will reach a peak and then decline to a much lower level. This process will be repeated as it becomes possible to diagnose more disorders, producing an increasing number of family groups for whom DNA testing is of diagnostic value. Once families have been tested with informative probes, then only the children born subsequently will require investigation so that a plateau in sample numbers will eventually be reached. It will be necessary to provide a safe repository for DNA samples, which may perhaps be stored for several generations, so that improved analysis can be carried out as new probes are developed. There are now probes available for use in about 20 serious diseases (covering nearly two thirds of the important single gene defects) any of which we might be asked to investigate.[1-4] Looking just at Huntington's disease, for which we now have 147 samples stored, in the Grampian region alone there are another 400–500 people who might require testing. There is a great deal of work for a molecular genetics laboratory, and we estimate that our present staff could cope with about 500 samples a year.

It is necessary to add to the range of probes maintained as research makes new cloned sequences available, but this also complicates estimates of costs. At present, a four probe, six polymorphism analysis of eight people might require consumables worth around £95 (estimated on the unit cost of enzyme, isotope, and hybridisation membrane), but mostly costs will vary depending on the sample load and the need to replace consumable materials. The time (10–12 days) taken to complete an analysis would be typical for other laboratories offering this kind of service.

For Aberdeen the consortium arrangement works well through cooperation and regular contact among staff in the four centres. Similar arrangements could undoubtedly be made in other areas so that expense was kept as low as possible, while allowing centres to develop skill in diagnosing a particular group of disorders. In Aberdeen introducing a molecular genetics laboratory has improved the service for patients and encouraged many new research initiatives of potential diagnostic value.

As the workload expands further problems will occur. Despite the experience of staff it may take a long time to convert research techniques into routine diagnostic use, although dedicated training courses could shorten this period. Inevitably, the priorities of the molecular genetics service will have to be determined, but cost benefit analysis of the existing molecular genetics service has already shown its value in patient care.[5] In the early years at least the numbers of medical and scientific staff may have to be increased with the growing number of disorders which can be analysed and as the families who are affected by genetic disease become aware of the power of the new technology.

References

1 Wetherall D. Molecular and cell biology in clinical medicine: introduction. *Br Med J* 1987; **295**: 587–9.
2 Pembrey M. Impact of molecular biology on clinical genetics. *Br Med J* 1987; **295**: 711–13.
3 Cooper D N, Schmidtke J. Diagnosis of genetic disease using recombinant DNA. *Hum Genet* 1986; **73**: 1–11.
4 Cooper D N, Schmidtke J. Diagnosis of genetic disease using recombinant DNA. *Hum Genet* 1987; **77**(suppl): 66–75.
5 Chapple J C, Dale R, Evans B G. The new genetics: will it pay its way? *Lancet* 1987; **i**: 1189–92.

Dictate a discharge summary

T M PENNEY

The main communication that a general practitioner receives about his or her patient's admission to hospital is the formal typed hospital discharge summary. This forms the core of available information and as such is of vital importance. Unfortunately, the task of dictating this summary is often regarded as a chore by the hospital doctor, which need not be the case if the job is tackled in a logical, systematic way.

At present there is a delay of about three weeks before the general practitioner receives the discharge summary.[1-3] The reasons for the delay are various but probably include delays in dictation and typing and postal delays.[1] If the summary can be dictated sooner, and in a way that requires the minimum of secretarial time, benefits will be reaped in several ways: the hospital doctor will enjoy up to date notes, the general practitioner will be aware of his or her patient's condition sooner, and the patients will be able to discuss their hospital stay and all its implications with their family doctor. Currently the system fails us.

I describe here how to dictate a discharge summary based on my own experiences and observations. I see no reason why most discharge summaries should not be received by the general practitioner within seven days of the patient's discharge if my guidelines are followed. With a standard format and better organisation the service can be vastly improved. It really is very easy to produce documents containing concise, relevant information if the right attitude to the task is adopted.

Design

I propose that all discharge summaries should be typed in one of

Dr Smith   Date
The Surgery
Anytown

Dear Dr Smith,

Re: Arthur BEST, 123 Anyroad, Anytown
Date of birth 1 2 34
Hospital No 567890

Admitted

Discharged

Diagnosis

History

Past medical history

Medication on admission

Examination

Investigations

Treatment and progress

Medication on discharge

Follow up

Yours sincerely,

Dr Jones,

Senior house officer to
Dr Brown, consultant

Fig. 1—*Standard discharge summary.*

two basic formats (figures 1 and 2). This would simplify the secretary's task and doctors would soon become accustomed to the
design, so minimising the chance of any important details being
omitted. Standard formats have been used successfully before.[4]

The short discharge letter may be used for any routine admission that is not complicated, when the general practitioner does
not need detailed information. It lends itself especially to patients
who have had operations and can be adapted to suit each particular
admission. To stick rigidly to a detailed format for a routine
appendicectomy, for example, wastes time and effort.

Dr Smith   Date
The Surgery
Anytown

Dear Dr Smith,

              Re: Arthur BEST, 123 Anyroad, Anytown
                     Date of birth 1 2 34
                     Hospital No 567890

      Your patient underwent a routine   operation
on   . There were no complications and he was discharged
on   , with the following medication: . Please
arrange for removal of stitches in   days. Follow up will not/will be
arranged for   weeks.

                        Yours sincerely,

                        Dr Jones,

                        Senior house officer to
                        Dr Brown, consultant

Fig 2—*Short discharge letter.*

For most admissions the standard discharge summary can be used. Some of the sections, however, could be omitted in certain cases—for instance, "Past medical history," "Medication on admission," and perhaps even "Examination" and "Investigations." The general practitioner does not really need to know that "there were signs of consolidation at the right base posteriorly and a consolidated area in the chest radiograph" if the diagnosis of pneumonia of the right lower lobe is written at the top of the page.

Details

The details written under each heading in the discharge summary should be concise and relevant. Strictly speaking, only details relevant to the general practitioner to whom the letter is addressed should be included. The copy of the summary left in the hospital notes, however, can be extremely useful to a subsequent admitting doctor because it acts as a précis of past events. For this reason some hospital practitioners will prefer, for instance, to give negative results of investigations as well as positive ones in the summary. I contend that to keep summaries as short as possible, and therefore save as much time as possible, such details should be omitted. It takes only a few seconds to turn to the investigation sheets in the hospital notes. A short, relevant, and concise summary is much more likely to be read through by a busy general practitioner than a long letter full of irrelevant material.

The most important headings for the general practitioner are "Diagnosis," "Medication on discharge," and "Follow up." In cases in which a new diagnosis has been made a few details under an additional heading of "Information given to the patient" would be invaluable. Awkward situations have arisen when patients have not been given vital pieces of information that the general practitioner has taken for granted and misunderstandings have subsequently occurred.

When each senior house officer takes up a new post the consultant should go over the system of discharge summaries used in the department and give initial guidance on the standards expected.

Dictation

Now that a standard format has been designed and the information condensed time must be found to dictate the summary. In my experience no specific time is set aside for a senior house officer to dictate summaries. The time must be found during the course of an already busy day, and this is often after everyone else has gone home. I well remember spending hours sitting alone in a darkened office, occasionally interrupted by the cleaner. Many senior house officers take their work home with them, although this is not wise because of the problems that arise concerning the security and confidentiality of patients' notes once they are taken outside the hospital.

Time should be made available every week—30 minutes should be sufficient—to dictate summaries. Perhaps the best time would be after the main ward round of the week, when decisions about discharging patients tend to be taken. Summaries could be dictated when the patients are sent home; the document will reach the general practitioner sooner, and the patients' individual details will be fresh in the mind of the senior house officer. Thus important details are less likely to be omitted and a better summary will be produced. If summaries are not dictated for several weeks it becomes more difficult to put a face to the patient's name. One has to thumb through notes to find the relevant information rather than being able to dictate most of the summary direct from memory.

I have experienced several disincentives to dictate summaries, the main one being a huge pile of notes overflowing from my pigeon hole in the consultant's office. A backlog develops surprisingly quickly, particularly at the start of a new hospital job. Often the senior house officer changes every six months, and the outgoing doctor may leave a residue of undictated notes behind. This is a dirty trick and quite unforgivable. The temptation would not be so great if dictation was performed promptly throughout the period of the job. Locums who do not dictate summaries on patients they look after present another problem; perhaps allocating the next senior member of the team to do the summaries while the senior house officer is away would help matters. A similar system could be adopted to cover holidays.

Equipment can also be a problem. Doctors should check that their dictaphones are recording properly and that their tapes are not damaged. I once came to the end of a long dictating session and checked the tape, only to find that the whole recording had been reduced to a series of unintelligible whirring and grinding noises.

Dispatch

After the summary has been dictated the tape should be labelled, attached to the notes, and left in a prearranged place for the secretary. Unfortunately, there is a general shortage of medical secretaries at present,[5] and typing may take several days or weeks. The senior house officer should make a habit of visiting the secretary's office regularly to sign the documents when they have been typed so that they may be posted without delay. Many hospitals use second class post.

References

1 Penney T M. Delayed communications between hospitals and general practitioners: where does the problem lie? *Br Med J* 1988; **297**: 28–9.
2 Mageean R J. Study of "discharge communications" from hospital. *Br Med J* 1986; **293**: 1283–4.
3 Tulloch A J, Fowler G H, McMillan J J, Spence J M. Hospital discharge reports: content and design. *Br Med J* 1975; **iv**: 443–6.
4 Stevenson J G, Murray Boyle C, Alexander W D. A new hospital discharge letter. *Lancet* 1973; **i**: 928–31.
5 Miller H C. Delayed communication between hospitals and general practitioners. *Br Med J* 1988; **297**: 292.

Write a practice annual report

STEFAN CEMBROWICZ

Our practice started producing an annual report five years ago. It began in a simple way, stimulated by an interest in recording the variety and volume of our work. It has now grown to fulfil a remarkable number of uses within and beyond the practice.

We operate a rotating medical editorship, with a different partner taking charge every year. Every doctor and each group of team members, including the cleaners, is "invited" to contribute and given a deadline of 1 January.

Our report starts with a foreword or introduction from a local personality or celebrity such as a councillor or the mayor or MP. This can be followed by an editorial review.

Structure of the practice and its team

Write a short background of the practice including a description of the premises and catchment area. Briefly describe the sort of records that are kept and whether you have a computer or word processor with specialised programmes. If necessary mention the communications available within the practice—whether bleeps, carphones, or hand held phones and which type of switchboard are used. Mention the range of publications in the practice library and list special practice equipment—for example, a video, resuscitation equipment, oxygen, nebulisers, electrocardiograph, and the facilities available for minor operation and family planning.

When you list the team members make it clear who are the principals, assistants, and trainees and to what extent locums and deputising services are used. The rest of the staff can then be included.

What to include in your annual report

Foreword or introduction
Editorial review
Description of practice—premises, equipment, staff, etc.
System of care provided
Audit
Finance
Reports from each group on the staff
Brickbats and bouquets
Illustrations, charts, photographs, poems

System of care

Under the heading "system of care" given the surgery hours for both the main surgery and branch surgeries. If specialist clinics are held, such as diabetic or well women clinics, these can be listed separately. This is a useful place to deal with your system for repeat prescriptions and any dispensing arrangements.

Audit

Audit is a fashionable concept these days and has an important place in any self respecting practice report. How this is laid down is a matter for individual preference.

Comparisons can be made between practice statistics and local, regional, and national figures such as attendance rates per patient and per year and patient turnover—that is, new patients and loss of patients because of death or moving away. Demographic details of the practice population should also include information on temporary residents. Much of this information can be relegated to the appendices.

It is worth having a section devoted to unusual aspects of the practice which could be a peculiarity of your catchment area and mention some particularly interesting patients who have been seen during the year. For instance, in our practice last year, the year of the Olympics, there were three cases of gynaecomastia among weightlifters who took illicit steroids.

Finance

It is important to provide information on the cost of the practice.

We include such items as the number of auxiliary staff per general practitioner and the costs per head of general practitioner services. It is illuminating to itemise prescribing costs from the Prescription Pricing Authority review and include the amounts of certain drugs prescribed such as benzodiazepines. Local and national comparisons are available, and we considered a "financial supplement" comparing our income from items of service payments with national averages. These figures can be gleaned from magazines such as *Medeconomics*.

Individual reports

In our health centre we have several dozen staff (including part timers), and we think that it is important for each staff group to have a say in the report. The brief is to define: (i) workload this year, (ii) aims for next year, and (iii) special problems.

We encourage collecting simple statistics and performance reviews. Many statistics are already collected by various team members but never gathered together.

Research, training, and teaching projects should be included, as well as papers that have been written. This might be followed by listing any outside sessions and other commitments such as occupational medicine or work for the Department of Health. Consider drawing a pie chart of the working day and saying how it could be improved. This is an ideal space for individual opinions to be aired, whether about special problems that have been experienced or ideas for the future.

A short piece on how study leave is used makes interesting reading, and perhaps you can finish off by naming the best medical book read during the year.

Layout and publishing

Keep the reader's attention by breaking up the pages with graphs, illustrations, pie charts, histograms, photographs—and even poems. Insert anecdotes, include some items on newsworthy local issues, and make use of a "brickbat and bouquet" section to publicise those who have caused problems or helped to solve them. Items from the waiting room suggestion box or comments from the patients' participation group add spice and ginger.

No one wants to read densely packed typewritten pages. Avoid solid blocks of type on the page; divide the pages into columns and use subheadings for each topic introduced. Some expert advice from an experienced journalist friend, relative, or patient can help you to avoid dull presentation. Copies of the *BMJ*, the *Lancet*, or even *Private Eye* are good examples of expert layouts.

Contributions should be typed on A4 paper and illustrations stuck down in the relevant places. Photocopy the whole lot and bind with plastic spines and a cardboard cover. One year a generous patient let us use his photocopier in exchange for a donation to charity.

Typing and making alterations on a word processor can produce a "letter quality" printout which can be photocopied commercially. This cost us £120 for 120 copies last year. The health authority or family practitioner committee may be able to help by allowing the use of their photocopying and collating equipment. This year the Royal College of General Practitioners charged £200 for producing 200 photocopies. Commercial printing would have cost a little more.

Colour snaps are relatively cheap to use for a team photograph, particularly if you use your High Street photo processing centre. One of these photos glued to the front cover makes it more likely that the report will be kept—at least by those in the picture.

Practices that have access to more up to date hardware can produce the layout with desktop publishing and use laser printing direct from a floppy disc.

This year we plan to insert an assessment slip into the report for readers to return to us with their comments.

Circulation list

The circulation list might include: all staff; friends and neighbouring practices; interested colleagues at home and abroad; members of trainers groups and research groups; the Royal College of General Practitioners; the regional adviser in general practice; the postgraduate tutor; local university departments of general practice; the district general manager; nursing officers and administrators; the community health council; the family practitioner committee; your MP.

Patients can be overlooked as a valuable resource to a practice so decide at an early stage whether you will give them access to a report, for instance, in the waiting room, on request, or through the patient participation group.

What it can achieve

Within the practice

Producing our annual report has been a painless introduction to simple performance review. This in turn has led to more detailed audit which has stimulated improved practice management—hesitant partners can be encouraged to contribute with the prospect of improved financial returns.

We find it a safe way of letting off steam as it airs issues that may not come to light during team or practice meetings. Visitors, students, trainees, and job applicants use it as a source of information, and we have found it useful as a reference store for projects and audits that may bear fruit in the years to come.

As a method of expressing common goals and tasks the report is invaluable and is a reminder that team members with widely differing backgrounds can share similar aims. As time goes by it is fascinating to read old copies and realise how much change there has been in the past five years, and it provides us all with a tangible record of the richness and diversity of general practice.

Outside the practice

As general practitioners working in a health centre we are aware that owing to shortages of cash the health authority is unable to maintain premises and supply staff in accordance with our original agreements. Mentioning these matters in a report which is widely circulated does seem to help.

I also find it is a way of keeping in touch and of exchanging ideas and enthusiasms with friends and neighbours whose practices may be greatly dissimilar from ours. Unpredictably, it can stimulate helpful suggestions from the most unexpected quarters. Doing a simple report is just another way of looking at the quality of care in practice and adding our support to the Royal College of General Practitioners' initiatives.

Standing back and looking at your work will help you to avoid being overwhelmed and burnt out by it and remind you of your rewards from it.

Don't be daunted by all this. A two page report may be more interesting than a 40 page report. Remember:

(1) Start small.
(2) Define your aims.
(3) Have a good look at someone else's report.
(4) Involve everybody.
(5) Enjoy doing it.

Be a GP locum

DAVID ALLEN STOCKS

"Our senior partner has collapsed. Can you take over, starting this evening?" Jobs are rarely arranged at such short notice, but when a doctor becomes "established" as a general practitioner locum the phone never stops ringing. Always keep a diary or calendar by the phone and pencil in the dates there and then. Have nothing to do with scraps of paper or the backs of envelopes: they float away into drawers and dustbins with important information lost forever. Double booking is the cardinal sin.

Becoming known

How does word get round that you are available for work? Try these methods:

Write to local general practitioners—I suggest sending a formal letter giving the dates when you are free. Enclose a copy of your curriculum vitae. A job might not be forthcoming but general practitioners like to have a pool of locums to draw from.

Write to your family practitioner committee—Family practitioner committees are not locum agencies, but they occasionally need a locum when a singlehanded GP is ill. The family practitioner committee may offer to send, for a fee, a copy of your curriculum vitae to each of the practices in its area.

Circulate at postgraduate meetings—Bump into your trainer, GP tutors, and former colleagues. This all helps to hang your name on the grapevine.

Enrol with agencies (but read the small print)—Local offices might be better than nationwide agencies. A doctor I know was asked to travel over 100 miles to do one afternoon's surgery. The BMA locum agency, administered from its regional offices, is free to members.

Advertise in medical journals—Give some flavour to your advertisement without sounding eccentric. Market yourself as a reliable and steady worker, neither bland nor spicy.

When responding to advertisements you must be quick off the mark: vacancies are soon filled.

The interview

Interviews are usually informal. They are thought of as introductions "to meet the other partners" or "to look round the health centre." The chit chat over coffee may be charming but don't be wrong footed into thinking the interview is a social call. You should be armed with your current certificates and copies of your curriculum vitae.

I am usually accepted at face value. My references have never been taken up, but it would be businesslike to ask your referees beforehand if they would mind giving your reference over the phone. Be sure of your dates before the interview. If you say "Yes, I'll definitely come" when offered the job then consider yourself caught: only illness or bereavement would let you comfortably off the hook.

Sort out pay and hours of work. You could accept the BMA guidelines on pay or use them as a basis for negotiation. There are standard rates for (*i*) a two hour surgery, (*ii*) a surgery and calls, and (*iii*) a full day. These are self explanatory, but if night or weekend work is required then make sure you know exactly what is expected. Also ask if the practice has any prescribing policies, such as antibiotics for sore throats. Try to comply with such policies without being a cipher. Ask for a timetable of your duties if the job lasts for longer than a day.

Before starting

When replacing a singlehanded GP phone the day before starting and ask about any seriously ill patients. I once called to see a patient without knowing that she was dying. The breezy tone of my visit was just wrong from the start. The patient looked disappointed. Her husband did not say much, but his expression seemed to say, "Our old doctor has left us in the lurch and sent this amateur instead." The quickest glance at the notes is better than nothing.

You will need drugs for emergency use and a bag for your equipment. You will have to pay for the drugs yourself, but they can be bought in small quantities from a pharmacist. Although tablets are readily available, drugs for injection are not always in stock; the pharmacist may need a day's notice to order them from the wholesale supplier. Controlled drugs are best kept in your pocket or bag and not in the car boot. A record of these drugs should be kept as they are bought and used.

If you intend to be a locum regularly then it is worth while buying a doctor's bag rather than making do with your battered old briefcase. Do pay attention to your appearance and "image"— patients like to size up the locum, so don't look like a ragbag even though you feel like a stopgap.

Your first day

Arrive five or 10 minutes early and ask to be shown round. Introduce yourself to the receptionists and the practice nurse. Ask for your name to be put on the door and find out where the doctor has gone on holiday—you will be asked this several times each surgery. Feel free to rearrange the furniture: I hate to use the desk as a defensive barrier. Find out if you shout or buzz for the first patient. If the corridor is not too long I like to go and collect each patient, although some regular attenders, primed for the buzzer, are unnerved by this little courtesy. Later in the day call in at the local pharmacy to introduce yourself.

Medical practice

As a locum I suffer from four temptations:

Superficiality—Patients who want to unburden an emotional problem will mostly prefer to consult a doctor they know. My locum work is biased towards acute minor illnesses. The temptation is to be superficial—to concentrate on the disease rather than the patient. This might suit most, but you should be alert to those patients with more deep rooted problems. When seeing a new doctor these patients often test the water first with a minor ailment before plunging in with an emotional disclosure.

Passing the buck—Not knowing the patients, you can easily fall behind appointment times, especially when these are at five minute intervals. I am then tempted to pass the buck: "Just take a few more of your tablets; they'll keep you going until your doctor comes back next week." You should do justice to the patient whose problem cannot be put off. Procrastination is a corruption of good medical practice.

Showing off—It is tempting to dazzle patients with a flash of brilliant plumage, and indeed a little knowledge can be finely dressed. But then the locum flies off, leaving the nest badly disturbed for the returning doctor. This particularly applies to those "heartsink" and difficult[2] patients who flatter you at their own doctor's expense. Similarly, regular prescriptions should not be changed merely for the sake of elegant variation: Still on those old tablets? I think these new ones will suit you much better. A locum should enjoy the tenancy but should leave things neat and tidy for the sitting tenant.

Lazy prescribing—In most practices the receptionist fills in the whole of the repeat prescription. All the doctor has to do is sign. Beware. Resist the importunity of harassed receptionists. Insist on seeing the notes first. Double check doses; treble check warfarin.[3] Be scrupulous with your signature; if in doubt, fail safe.

Visits

For visits you will need a map, a *British National Formulary*, the phone numbers of hospitals and ambulance control, and plenty of headed notepaper and prescriptions. An experienced receptionist will put the non-urgent visits in order so that you can drive a circular tour. Ask for the patients' phone numbers to be written on the front of the notes. Inner city visits are a nightmare for the stranger: flyovers and one way streets, underpasses, and no parking signs all conspire against you. Never be tempted on to an urban motorway. Street signs have been pulled down and house numbers have been painted over. Don't despair. Country visits, too, have their pleasures: roads dwindle into dirt tracks, houses hide behind trees. If you are seriously lost ring the local police. When visiting at night ask for all the lights to be switched on and for the curtains to be left open.

Playing fair

Most surgeries last for about two hours. Locums are not paid to the minute, so keep working with a good grace if you are still busy after two and a half hours: tomorrow's surgery might last for only an hour and 40 minutes.

All the GPs I have worked for have been honourable employers, but watch out for a nominal one hour surgery, paid at half of the two hour rate, that regularly lasts all morning.

A sharp practice is to find yourself replacing two doctors. If you are overwhelmed with work speak to the senior partner or the practice manager. Do this before cracking up.

Write in the notes as carefully as possible. Abandon your darling shorthand and stick to standard abbreviations. Write legibly or not at all—the medical secretary is a suitable judge.

If the GP you are replacing refers patients to a particular consultant in each specialty then try to follow suit.

One or two patients will ask for a second opinion from you. A niggling dissatisfaction with their GP is often apparent. The patient's interests come first, of course, so the symptoms and signs must be assessed impartially, but it is unprofessional to erode any further the patient's confidence in the doctor. I believe that polite neutrality is the best response when patients criticise their GP. Listening carefully to the patient might be enough to soothe the irritation.[4]

Frustrations and rewards

A few patients will be disappointed about not seeing their usual doctor. The hurt tone of "Where's *the* doctor?" says it all. Don't be discouraged. One day patients might become as loyal to you. Occasionally a patient will refuse to be examined. I used to be upset by this, but now I simply ask the patient to return either the following day or within a week. If the symptoms sound serious then leave a note for the doctor when you leave.

Not being able to follow up patients is frustrating, especially when you suspect some unusual disease. I sometimes call in several weeks after leaving a surgery to inquire about such patients.

Locum general practice is ideal work for a doctor looking for a permanent GP job. One picks up so many ideas for the perfect practice, including things to avoid. Practices are like the suburbs of London: some are up and coming, some are fashionable, and some have seen better days. Surgery accommodation varies from the palatial to the poky. But patients everywhere deserve the best.

There is satisfaction in trying to practise a high standard of medicine for every patient irrespective of surroundings.

References

1 O'Dowd T C. Five years of heartsink patients in general practice. *Br Med J* 1988; **297**: 528–30.
2 Gerrard T J, Riddell J D. Difficult patients: black holes and secrets. *Br Med J* 1988: **297**; 530–2.
3 Medical Defence Union. *Annual report.* London: MDU, 1988; 40.
4 Calnan J. *Talking with patients.* London: Heinemann, 1983.

Develop diabetic care in general practice

R L GIBBINS, J SAUNDERS

It is generally accepted that the quality of care provided for people with diabetes can be considerably improved, both in general practice and in hospital clinics. Although we concentrate here on general practice, there must be a cooperative arrangement between the generalist and the specialist, each with defined areas of responsibility if a good standard of care is to come about.

The division of responsibility will depend heavily on local factors such as what is available in the diabetic clinic and what skills general practitioners already have or can learn. The needs of different geographic areas will also vary. The final decision on what system of care is used in a practice must rest with the general practitioners since they have the responsibility of ensuring that it works.

What follows is based on our experience in a rural area of mid-Wales, with practices centred on small towns, some with general practitioner hospitals, and served by district hospitals some of which are up to 40 miles away.

Staged approach to improving care

Tackling the problem head on is a daunting prospect, and we found that a staged approach minimised the potential trauma. The stages were as follows: (*a*) Produce a register of all known patients with diabetes in the practice. (*b*) Do a baseline survey of the current state of these patients. (*c*) Then identify areas where improvement is necessary and agree a practice protocol for diabetic care. (*d*) Implement a system of recall and clinical review for diabetic patients. (*e*) At regular intervals thereafter repeat the initial survey of care to identify any problem areas and evaluate the exercise.

In a busy practice the elements of this plan that are most likely to be omitted are the baseline and follow up surveys because of the amount of work entailed. Diabetic care in the practice is likely to improve without them, but it will not be possible to quantify the improvement or identify those areas in which problems remain.

Producing a register

Producing a register of diabetic patients in the practice will require little of the doctors' time. The receptionists and practice staff are asked to record all patients who receive repeat prescriptions for insulin, hypoglycaemic drugs, or testing sticks. Everybody in the practice tries to remember which patients have diabetes; the local diabetic clinic can be asked for a list of patients from the practice who attend, though this information may not be available. If there is sufficient demand, however, it should become available.

For each diabetic patient identified a small card is made out, recording the patient's name, address, sex, general practitioner's name, type of treatment, and the date the patient was last seen. The cards are stored in alphabetical order using a card index, and patients' notes are tagged with a coloured sticker. This process of collecting patients needs to continue for at least three months, by which time the number identified should approach 1% of the practice population. The register should, however, be kept "open" indefinitely. In our experience the initial 1% may increase to 2% by three years.

Baseline survey

One doctor at least has to become more involved when the baseline survey is carried out. The practice must agree a set of data to be collected, which may include some demographic and epidemiological items. We used the following items: (a) Sex, date of birth (or age), age at diagnosis, and type of treatment for each patient. (b) Date last seen by general practitioner for diabetic care; date last seen in consultant clinic for diabetic care. (c) The date previous to the survey date that the following criteria were recorded in the notes: weight; blood pressure, concentrations of blood glucose, glycated haemoglobin, and blood urea or creatinine; visual acuity.

(d) The date previous to the survey date that the feet and eyes were examined and fundoscopy results categorised as normal, background change, maculopathy, proliferative retinopathy, or other non-diabetic disease such as cararact.

Unless you are familiar with computers the easiest way of recording this information is in tabular form with a line for each patient and columns for the data.

This mass of information must then be analysed. This potentially alarming stage can be quite simple. The numbers of diabetics who take insulin, oral agents, and are being treated with diet alone are compared with the total number of patients in the practice to give a rough prevalence (or ascertainment rate) for the separate groups and overall. The sex distribution and the mean age at the survey date and at diagnosis can also be calculated. The numbers of patients in each group and overall seen by their general practitioner within six months, 12 months, over 12 months, and never are counted to give an estimate of the frequency of contact with the general practitioner. A similar assessment of contact with consultants is made using time intervals of 12 months, 24 months, over 24 months, and never.

For weight and blood glucose concentration the percentages recorded within six months are calculated. For blood pressure, glycated haemoglobin, visual acuity, fundoscopy, and foot examination the percentages recorded within 12 months are calculated, and for urea or creatinine concentration the percentage within five years is calculated. The means and standard deviations for each group can be analysed to give an estimate of overall control of diabetes and the percentage in each category for eye examination results calculated.

Discussing results, agreeing a practice protocol

Collecting data is made much simpler if the patients' notes are organised in chronological order, and these should include results from consultant clinic letters. If there is a suitably trained or enthusiastic member of the practice staff much of the collection and analysis of data can be delegated. The information then needs to be typed up and circulated round the practice, preferably to attached nursing staff as well, who may have an important role later on. The local consultant in diabetes might be interested in seeing a copy, provided the results are not too embarrassing.

Holding a practice meeting might be the best way to decide what to do in the light of the results. In our case the results were not good, nor were they in any of the seven other practices that reached this stage. Although three quarters of the patients were being seen by their general practitioner at less than six monthly intervals, routine recording of basic data was not being done.

Because of this most of the practices concerned have developed a recall and review system for their diabetic patients. At this stage it seems reasonable to suggest a framework around which a practice protocol could be produced.

Expected quality of care

This protocol, arrived at by discussion between general practitioners and the consultant, sets the basic standard for both general practitioner and hospital care in terms of clinical measurement. The division of responsibility for specific items will need defining for each practice depending on available skills. Which types of patients will be looked after by general practitioners also needs defining but should include most of those who are not taking insulin and many insulin takers who have uncomplicated disease.

When the patient is first seen a general history should be taken and an examination carried out and all data for the yearly assessment (see below) measured. In addition, the patient's height should be measured and ideal body weight or body mass index calculated, and blood urea or creatinine concentration measured to assess renal function. Follow up visits should be made at six month intervals and no longer.

The six monthly assessment should include at least a measurement of weight, urine analysis for protein and ketones, blood glucose concentration (preferably after an interval since food was last taken), and details of treatment and time of the next visit.

The yearly assessment should include all the data for the six monthly assessment, and blood pressure, glycated haemoglobin concentration, visual acuity (corrected if necessary), fundoscopy with dilated pupils (preferably in a darkened room), and a check on skin condition, peripheral pulses, and reflexes especially in the legs.

Every five years renal function should be assessed by checking blood urea or creatinine concentrations.

Devising a system of recall

By now the practice should have agreed the frequency and content of consultation. There must be enough flexibility in the system for variations from the norm for some patients. For example, those whose diabetes has recently been diagnosed and those in whom control is poor will need to consult more often. The next requirement is a system for regularly recalling the patients or at least recording when they were last seen.

The simplest way of doing this is to use the pre-existing card index of diabetic patients. The cards that were originally filed in alphabetical order are divided into six equal groups, assuming a maximum recall interval of six months. If, for instance, the recall system is to start in January the cards are then filed under the calendar months January to June, leaving July to December free. The group who are to be seen in January are sent for, and when they attend their cards are refiled in whatever month the doctor decides they shoud next be seen. The cards for those who do not attend can be refiled for further appointments in February or March. The recall index takes about a year to sort itself out, but by then roughly equal numbers of patients should be coming in each month. The cards of those who are excluded from the recall system can be filed separately. An alternative way of starting the recall system is to send for patients in their month of birth, though this is more suited to a yearly than a six monthly review.

If you have a computer there should be a recall facility in all software packages for general practice, though these are usually incapable of storing numerical data unless previously encoded. It is advisable to have a manual backup as relatively minor typographical errors may "lose" a patient in a computer database, and interruptions of electrical supply or malfunctions in hardware may lose them all.

We then use a separate card to record the patients' visits. There are several available, some from pharmaceutical companies. We modelled ours on the antenatal cooperation card, putting the additional information collected at the first visit on the front cover. Inside are columns for weight, urine analysis, blood glucose and glycated haemoglobin concentrations, two larger spaces for less frequent tests such as eye and foot examination, and space for details of management. In a final column the interval to the next visit is recorded. Folded in half, this card fits into a Lloyd George envelope, though we keep them separately. The card should be kept simple, otherwise there is a danger that it will not be completely filled in. The card can be given to the patient and used by both general practitioners and the hospital clinic for patients who attend both. This would require discussion with the consultants concerned. If the practice produces its own card the local branch of the British Diabetic Association might help with the cost.

Review process

One fear expressed by several practices was that the workload might be greater. For the doctors this would mean more consultation time. But this can be minimised by the participation of attached nursing staff. Nurses are generally better trained in the repetitive tasks of measuring height, blood pressure, etc, than doctors and are more reliable at recording them. Many patients may find it easier to see a nurse as the first contact for problems with their diabetes, and the nurse is well placed to provide patient education, which is essential. The doctor should do more complex clinical tests, assess the basic information collected by the nurse, and decide on necessary changes in management. The doctor can also arrange referrals to paramedical services such as dietitians, chiropodists, ophthalmic opticians (with whom it may be possible to arrange yearly eye examinations), and consultant clinics. Needless to say, direct referral from general practice to all these services must be available. This is especially true of dietitians as most of the patients who do not take insulin will be cared for in general practice, and many of these should need only dietary advice to achieve adequate control of their diabetes. In addition, the general practitioner bears overall clinical responsibility for the patient and must coordinate and manage the whole system.

Patients may be seen in various ways. Partners may see their own patients, or one doctor may see all the diabetics, perhaps in clinics held weekly or monthly. If the practice has an appointment system patients may be given concurrent appointments with the nurse and doctor. Whatever method is chosen it must fit in with other practice routines and will vary from practice to practice. Our system depends heavily on an enthusiastic nurse, who sees patients first, weighs them, measures blood glucose concentrations, blood pressure, and visual acuity, checks their feet, takes blood for glycated haemoglobin, and dilates the pupils (thus ensuring the fundi are examined) before patients are seen by their own doctor. She also gives advice on prevention and organises patient education. The essential feature is that protected time of some sort is given to the patient.

It is essential to train nursing staff for this type of work. Although formal training may be available for hospital based diabetes liaison sisters, this may not be suitable for nurses in primary care. We found that making arrangements with the local consultant unit was adequate. It may also be advisable for one of the doctors to attend a refresher course.

Each practice will develop a different pattern of care depending on the facilities available in their area, and the above picture is only given as an example. For those working in health centres where ophthalmic opticians also attend there is a good opportunity for arranging yearly eye examinations using the diabetic register. We do not have this facility, and eye surveillance is a problem area for us, though as we examine fundi more regularly we inevitably get better at it. With practice all doctors should be capable of deciding whether a fundus is normal or abnormal; if an abnormality is seen or suspected there must be rapid access to a specialist opinion. This is one area in which specialist departments can help by organising refresher courses for general practitioners.

Whatever system is devised it is useful to know whether it is working, which requires a regular audit. This can be a repeat of the baseline survey, and a sensible interval is every two years. At this point it is helpful to have a suitable computer system.

How well does it work?

The system needs to operate for at least a year, and preferably two, before improvement can be assessed. This is done by repeating the baseline survey, much of which may again be delegated. Our practice and one other have done this, mainly from the point of view of frequency of surveillance rather than quality of control, since this seemed the first priority. Results are very encouraging, with a dramatic improvement in all the criteria measured. The patients have expressed their appreciation, too. Default rates are very low, which may reflect the prescribing power of general practitioners. It remains to be seen whether this leads to improved control of diabetes. In future surveys we hope to have enough paired data on individual patients to begin to answer this question.

We thank all the health workers concerned, especially the Bulith Wells and Brecon Medical Group Practices, and the Neville Hall Hospital Thrombosis and General Research Fund and the Claire Wand Fund for financial support.

Useful reading

Alberti K G M M, Hockaday T D R. Diabetes mellitus. In: *Oxford textbook of medicine*. Vol 1. Oxford: Oxford University Press, 1983; 5–48.

British Diabetes Association, 10 Queen Anne Street, London W1M 0BD (for information).

Howie J G R. *Research in general practice*. London: Croom Helm, 1979.

Sonksen P, Fox C, Judd S. *The diabetes reference book*. London: Harper and Row, 1985.

Watkins P J. *ABC of diabetes*. London: British Medical Association, 1983.

Start and run a medical dining club

J H BARON

British medicine has many curious customs. One of the least known and most idiosyncratic is the Dining Club. A club can be scientific, semiscientific, or simply sybaritic. I explain here the origin of these clubs and give detailed advice on how to start one and run it successfully. I do not cover alumni or surgical travelling clubs: they present no problems. Nor do I discuss groups such as the Breathing Club, whose members respire and cerebrate, but neither eat nor drink.

History

Most of our famous professional societies began as a small group of friends with a common interest, who discussed, drank, and dined together regularly: Aubrey's "sodality in a tavern", or Dr Johnson's "an assembly of good fellows meeting under certain conditions". With a small membership renewed only on resignation or death such clubs may survive for centuries. Once the membership of the club expands into hundreds or thousands with the advance of the particular specialty, then the members cannot all dine together intimately. There is then a need for a club within a club and a new small fraction of the larger society comes together to meet, drink, and dine with one another. Thus the British Society of Gastroenterology began with 39 members in 1937 but now has 1500, so that on the evening before its annual dinner smaller groups meet, each with its own theme.

Clubs go back three centuries. Robert Boyle's Invisible College of experimental philosophers met weekly from 1645, often in the Bull's Head Tavern in Cheapside. By 1648 it had a satellite, the

Philosophical Society of Oxford, a 30 member Greate Clubbe. In 1660 these two amalgamated to become the Royal Society, with 55 members, now grown to 1105.

After the Wednesday meetings groups of Fellows supped at different taverns, such as the Crowne Taverne Club, the Club at the Sun, Halley's Club and the Virtuosoe's Club at Jonathan's Tavern in Cornhill. The records of the present Royal Society Club[1][2] date from 1743, with eight members dining on fish and pudding with porter for half a crown (12.5p).[1][2] Membership increased to 40 in 1748, 66 in 1900, and later 75. The club now meets for dinner twice a year, with no formal business except the toast to the "arts and sciences". At its 7573rd dinner in 1974 it was agreed that women should be granted membership.

Menu of the Royal Society Club

24 March 1747

Fresh Salmon   Lobster Sauce
Cods Head
Pidgeon Pye
Calves Head
Bacon & Greens
Fillett of Veal
Chine of Pork
Plumb Pudding
Apple Custard
Butter & Cheese

Fig 1—*Menu of the Royal Society Club*,[2] *24 March 1747.*[8]

A group of scientists and technologists in Birmingham met together in 1757 and became a formal circle in 1766. Dinner at Matthew Boulton's house was always followed by scientific discussion. This Lunar Society met every full moon for ease of travelling at night. Engineers started to dine on Friday evenings in 1771 at the King's Head Tavern before forming the Smeatonian Society of Civil Engineers. The Society of Antiquaries started their dining club in 1774. The Royal Society of Edinburgh, founded in 1783, had its own Club from 1820, and others briefly (New Club 1832–40, Supper Club 1834–5).[3]

Of the social clubs who have their own buildings, the oldest is White's (1693), and there are several others of the mid-eighteenth century, such as Brook's (1746) and Boodle's (1762). Dining clubs, however, usually began in taverns, such as the Dilettanti (1732), now meeting at Brook's, or the artist-governors of the Foundling Hospital (1746), the forerunners of the Royal Academy of 1768. Dr Johnson and Sir Joshua Reynolds founded the Literary Club in 1764 with nine members dining each Monday at 7 pm at the Turk's Head.[4]

The Royal College of Physicians of London had at least two dining clubs, the younger of which was founded before 1764. They merged in 1834 and were still going strong in 1909.[5] Many of the early minute books of these clubs have not survived. The early records of the Medical Club, afterwards known as the Sydenham Club, are said to have been stolen by a footpad from one of the first secretaries walking home across the park, but their account books date from 1796. Wagers were common—for example, in 1854, "that Miss Nightingale is not married by the next meeting", and "that Miss Nightingale has a child by this day twelve month".[6] The club still numbers 18, six each of physicians, surgeons, and "apothecaries." The St Alban's Medical Club, named after the tavern where it first met, has records dating back to 1789.[7] It now has seven each of physicians, surgeons, and apothecaries, dines three times a year, and has occasionally dined together with its old rival the Sydenham Club.

Several other clubs have mixed family doctor or specialist membership. The Chelsea Clinical Society was founded in 1896 with nine members for informal discussion about medical problems: "whisky should be provided, but no women."[8] By 1910 there were over 100 members, and formal, clinical, and pathological presentations and volumes of published proceedings. It now has 300 members dining formally (with spouses) five times a year. The Hunterian goes back to 1819 and now has 500 members with 10 dinners a year, as well as the Hunterian Oration at the Royal College of Surgeons.

Some clubs are confined to a particular city or specialty. Thus Oxford has the Circle of Willis (1920s) and the breakaway Bundle of His (1966): each dines every term. Cambridge has the Carphologists Club, and Edinburgh has the Aesculapian Club (1773) with 11 FRCP and 11 FRCS members dining twice a year. Other clubs in Edinburgh are the Royal Medico-Chirurgical, the Coulston, and the Harveian. General practitioners just south of Hyde Park formed a Sloane Medical Society in 1973. Among the Orthopaedic Clubs are the Girdlestone, Lippman-Kessel, Arbuthnot Lane, Percival Pott, Sesamoid, Innominate and Nibblers, some of which were started by peer groups of trainees who continue to meet once or twice a year to discuss clinicopathological problems, followed by dinner with spouses.

One medical club was started by the government. After the 1914–18 war the Ministry of Pensions was faced with major economic pressures from those said to be disabled from heart disease. In 1920 the ministry appointed regional cardiological advisers who also met in committee in London from time to time. In 1922 John Cowan turned this group into a 15 member Cardiac Club which became the British Cardiac Society in 1937.[9][10]

The Dublin Biological Club was founded in Trinity College Dublin in 1872 "to consider the morbid and healthy conditions of animal and vegetable life".[11][12] Members originally numbered 14, then 18, and later 30. The club met weekly from October to June, and each member had to present a paper at least once a year. Refreshment was at first limited to light ale, but later there were annual dinners, followed by kite-flying, quoits, and firing with .22 bore rifles at empty champagne bottles.

Carte de Vins	
Old Chablis	Huêtres au Citron
Milk Punch	Tortue claire Tortue liée
Madeira (1857)	Saumon de Christchurch
Johannisberg (1862)	Blanchailles
Perrier Jouet	Ris de Veau à la Montpensier
(1874)	Chaud-froid de Cailles à la St James
Amontillado	Selle de Mouton de Galles
Chateau Lafitte	Selle d'Agneau de Sussex
(1875)	Petits Canetons rôtis
Martinez Port	Petits Pois
(1865)	Asperges en Branches, Sauce Mousseline
Boulestin's Cognac	Pouding à la Burlington
(1810)	Tarte aux Pommes
Kümmel	Pailles au Parmesan
Café	Dessert

Fig 2—*Menu of the College Club, Burlington Hotel, 22 February 1897, when the Prince of Wales dined.*[5]

167

Most clubs last only for the active lives of their founders and then are forgotten in the absence of any surviving papers. Fortunately, one is documented.[13] The Hexagon Club was founded for six neurologists by Sir Charles Symonds at a dinner at his Wimpole Street home on 30 April 1930 with Russell Brain, Hugh Cairns, Macdonald Critchley, Derek Denny-Brown, and George Riddoch. All were connected with the National Hospital for Nervous Diseases, Queens Square. They chose to meet regularly at a neutral site, the Great Central Hotel. Conversation was general before and during the dinner, but after dinner at each meeting one member (in turn alphabetically) gave a 20 to 30 minute paper followed by a fierce discussion. Many of these papers, much improved by this rehearsal, appeared in *Brain*; others disappeared without trace. The club occasionally had foreign guests—Foerster (1931, 1932), Lhermitte (1934), and Broewer (1936). The club ended when World War II broke out.

Conclusion

If you work in an exciting new field and want to talk freely in a congenial ambience with a few colleagues, then consider starting a medical dining club. Find an equally gregarious and obsessional friend to help: the more literate of the two can become secretary, the more numerate treasurer. Then write round to suitable prospective members to come to a dinner to discuss your proposal and the future is yours. The following appendices may help.

Appendix 1–Model rules for a semiscientific club

1 *Name*—This association shall be called the Navel Club in honour of Sir Nathaniel Navel, 1750–1851.

2 *Object*—This club is constituted to provide opportunities for those interested in the secretions of the umbilicus to meet for discussion and fellowship.

3 *Meetings*—The club will hold at least one, and as many meetings each year as the committee decide. Meetings will usually be held on the evening before the annual meeting of the British Society of Omphalology. Each meeting will consist of a dinner, of which members will be given due notice by the secretary so that they can pay the treasurer in advance if they

are attending. Members may bring to the dinner, by prior notification, guests interested in the secretions of the umbilicus. Speakers and topics for discussion will be decided by the committee.

4 *Ordinary membership*—Persons domiciled in Britain with a major interest in the secretions of the umbilicus are eligible for ordinary membership of the club. Founder members will be selected at a foundation meeting. Additional members may be elected at any meeting of the club after prior notice to the secretary with the candidate's name and umbilical interest and with the signatures of a proposer and seconder. Ordinary membership is limited to 50.

5 *Senior members*—Ordinary members automatically become senior members on their 65th birthday.

6 *Honorary membership*—The club may elect to honorary membership those ineligible to ordinary membership because of domicile abroad. Honorary members have all the privileges of membership but shall not pay a subscription.

7 *Corresponding members*—Ordinary members who take up domicile abroad automatically become corresponding members with all the privileges of membership.

8 *Subscription*—On election each member shall pay to the treasurer a life subscription of £5.00.

9 *Finance*—The club shall be financed by contributions from its members. Grants from other organisations and donations from persons desiring to support the club shall be accepted at the discretion of the committee.

10 *Management*—The business of the club shall be conducted by the committee, which will have sole control in all matters relating to the club. The committee shall consist of the president, the secretary, the treasurer, and two additional members. Two members of the committee shall constitute a quorum.

11 *Election of officers*—The president shall be elected annually and is not eligible for reappointment. The secretary and treasurer should be elected annually and be eligible for reappointment. The two other members of the committee shall serve for three years and shall not be eligible for immediate reappointment.

12 *General meetings*—The club will hold an inaugural meeting to draw up the rules of the society, and thereafter shall hold an annual general meeting at which 10 members shall constitute

a quorum. At the annual general meeting reports of the treasurer and secretary shall be presented and the officers elected.

13 *Amendments to rules*—The rules of the club can be amended at any annual general meeting when notice of proposed changes has been given to each member at least two weeks previously. No changes shall be made unless two thirds of the voting membership are in favour.

Notes

Rule 1—A constitution is essential for any club, if only to satisfy a bank manager on opening an account.

Rule 2—Ensure that members pay in advance. A scientific or even a semiscientific club should have a theme to each dinner, either a discussion paper by a member or guest or a debate carefully argued by a proposer and an opposer on a topic made known to the membership in the annual notice. A toast to "The Queen" can be followed by one in honour of the founder: "The Memory of Nathaniel Navel." This provides an opportunity for some historical references to the development of omphalology in the city in which the club is dining, or the country of origin or domicile of the guest of honour, with some appropriate remarks on the life and times of the founder.

Rule 4—Do not have ordinary members from abroad. Scientific or semiscientific societies should not blackball new members, and in practice it is advisable for the committee to recommend to the postprandial annual general meeting candidates to fill vacancies arising from death, resignation, emigration, or seniority. Members need not come every year: it is more enjoyable and intimate if they do not so that the members, including guests, are less than 40. Members who stop coming usually resign voluntarily, or can be so persuaded.

Rule 6—Limit honorary membership to those from overseas, usually one each year, and avoid the invidious task of selecting Britons for honours.

Rule 8—The club finances itself from the monies gained from dinners, but needs a small working capital obtained from an entry fee, which avoids the effort and expense of collecting annual subscriptions.

Rule 9—Clubs are often offered hospitality by industry. The committee should consider carefully whether doctors should dine at the expense of others.

Rule 10—The business of the club can usually be managed by the secretary in, say, 10 hours a year. The committee need never meet, but its members can be asked by post to nominate the next president, guest of honour, new members, topics and debaters. The secretary and the treasurer should stay for years if they are efficient but must be subject to formal reappointment each year.

Appendix 2—Model rules for a sybaritic club

1 The club shall be called the Sir Lancelot Spratt Dining Club.
2 It shall be limited to 15 members who shall be proposed and elected by the members.
3 It shall hold not less than one dinner each year, at which members will preside in rotation.
4 One member shall be elected as president for one year only; another shall be elected as secretary/treasurer for one year and be eligible for re-election. The secretary shall keep the minutes, incorporating the menu of the dinner and the signatures of the members present.
5 A member absent over two consecutive years shall be deemed to have offered his or her resignation.
6 Members attaining the age of 70 years (or 65) shall become senior members and will not be counted within the limits of 15 members of the club, nor will they be liable to forced resignation under rule 5.
7 Each member may propose one name for any vacancy. The secretary shall send a list of such proposals to all members, who shall record their vote(s) according to the number of vacancies and return the ballot paper to the secretary. A member may vote against any name on the list by striking it out, and one such adverse vote shall exclude that proposal. A second ballot shall then take place on those proposals which scored most votes on the first ballot, and the list on the second ballot should contain one more name than the number of vacancies. This list should be circulated to all members to vote as before, but no name can be excluded on the second or subsequent ballot. Any problems in election shall be solved at the next club dinner under the direction of the president, who shall have a casting vote.

8   Any changes to the rules shall be forwarded to the secretary, proposed and seconded, so that a postal ballot can be conducted with two thirds of the membership being necessary for the change to be agreed.

Notes

Rule 2—A sybaritic dining club must be small enough to dine around one table, about six to 18 in number.

Rule 3—Most clubs dine annually and some three or four times a year.

Rule 4—The president should be changed annually. The secretary should remain in post for years.

Rule 5—A small closely knit club does not want members who come only occasionally. Their membership should be deemed to have lapsed after their absence for two consecutive years.

Rule 6—Older members may find it difficult to come each year and should be encouraged to come whenever they can.

Rule 7—New members must be acceptable to everyone else, and most clubs operate a "one blackball excludes" rule. Some are more tolerant and two blackballs are needed as veto.

References

1   Geikie R A. *Royal Society Club. The record of a London dining club in the eighteenth and nineteenth centuries*. London: Macmillan, 1917.
2   Allibone T E. *The Royal Society and its dining clubs*. Oxford: Pergamon, 1976.
3   Guthrie D. *A short history of the Royal Society Club of Edinburgh 1820–1962*. Edinburgh: (privately printed), 1962.
4   Murdoch T. Talk of the Town. *Country Life* 1988; **182**: 180–1.
5   Payne J F. *History of the College Club of the Royal College of Physicians of London*. London: (privately printed), 1909.
6   Wellcome Institute for the History of Medicine. The Medical Club. In: *A vision of history*. London: The Wellcome Trust, 1986; 24.
7   Price R. St Albans Medical Club. *J Internat Wine Food Soc* 1979; **6**: 7–17.
8   Harvey W. *A History of the Chelsea Clinical Society*. London: (privately printed), 1962.
9   Cowan J. Some notes on the Cardiac Club. *Br Heart J* 1939; **1**: 97–104.
10   Campbell M. The British Cardiac Society and Cardiac Club: 1922–61. *Br Heart J* 1962; **24**: 673–95.
11   Bewley G. An account of the Biological Club. *Irish J Med Sci* 1960; **409**: 1–15.
12   Foot A W. Reminiscences of the Dublin Biological Club. *Dublin J Med Sci* 1892; **93**: 425–41.
13   Critchley M. Posthumous papers of the Hexagon Club. In: *The Citadel of the senses and other essays*. New York: Raven Press, 1985; 109–20.

Commission a portrait

IMOGEN SHEERAN

For many of us the prospect of having our portrait painted is quite daunting. There may be no choice in the matter if the portrait has been commissioned by an outside body to commemorate your life's achievements. Even if you are a willing participant commissioning a portrait for yourself the process must be carefully considered. The past decade has seen a tremendous upsurge in interest in all types of figurative art, and portraiture especially has been given a new impetus. The resultant wide choice of artists and styles makes the task of commissioning both more simple and more complex. No longer limited to a formulaic photographic likeness or "society" portrait, you may choose a style of painting and format to suit your mood and budget. You might want to commission an established portraitist whose clients may range from academics and aesthetes to pop stars and politicians. Or you might be more adventurous and seek out young talent from an art school's diploma show or tailor made exhibition such as the annual John Player Portrait Award for portrait painters under 40.

Points to consider when commissioning a portrait

- Type of artist—young inexperienced, experimental, established, fashionable
- Medium—oil, acrylic, pastel, watercolour, drawing, mixed media, sculpture, photograph
- Size and format—full length, three quarter length, half length, head and shoulders, miniature, lifesize, full face, three quarter face, profile
- Style—photographic likeness *v* artistic licence
- Setting and dress—home, office, studio; academic gown, informal, iconography, association

---

There are two overriding considerations in commissioning a portrait. What is it for and how much can it cost? Purpose and budget will affect all other criteria. Is it a formal portrait to be placed alongside those of fellow worthies? Or a private commission to display at home, intended to record your personality not status? Have you a free reign in the choice of medium, size, format, and style? Or are these dictated by the nature of the commission? Is the portrait part of an existing series to which it must conform? Will your budget cover the considerable costs of an established society portrait painter or would you prefer to test younger talent or a more experimental artist?

Homework

Having a portrait made is quite an undertaking in terms of both time and money so you must do adequate homework to ensure the smooth running of the venture. This begins well away from the artist's studio in your acquiring a grounding in portraiture. Visit a number of exhibitions in which portraits are included and take a historical overview at the National Portrait Gallery. Looking closely at historic and contemporary portraits helps an educated approach to your chosen artist and will also help you decide on the right format. Specialist exhibitions include the annual John Player Portrait Award at the National Portrait Gallery and the Royal Society of Portrait Painters' annual exhibition, both of which show a wide spectrum of contemporary work. Photographic dossiers on many portrait artists are kept at the National Portrait Gallery, the Royal Society of Portrait Painters, and at other specialist galleries such as the New Grafton Gallery, London. These can be examined by appointment.

Points to consider when budgeting for a portrait

- Trips to exhibitions, artists, previous patrons
- First sitting, subsequent sittings
- Studies, maquettes
- Finished portrait
- Varnishing, glazing, framing, casting, mounting, unveiling or exhibiting, lighting, hanging, entertainment

---

After viewing exhibitions and photographic records you should have some idea of whose work you would like to see in detail. It is important not only to visit the artists themselves but also to view collections of their work and to talk to previous sitters about their experiences and misgivings. During informal studio visits you should discuss your expectations for your commission. What do you want from the portrait—mere likeness (in which case why not have a photograph taken instead) or a record of past achievements? Do you wish to include professional or personal iconography? What kind of setting had you envisaged? Whether there is empathy between you or a personality clash will soon become apparent, an important consideration as the portrait making process can be quite intense and exposing.

Sorting out the details

Once you have found a sympathetic artist whose work you admire you must have another more formal meeting to discuss the contract, budget, and timescale. How many sittings will there be? What happens if one of you have to withdraw because of other commitments? What happens if the first sitting or subsequently finished portrait is not acceptable. Which stages of the commission require payment? Some artists make no charge for the preliminary sitting and sketches. Others will not charge if you reject the finished portrait. You are most unlikely to do so as they will usually agree to alter or repaint the work. Your contract is a "gentleman's agreement" not a legal document—all the artist has to do is supply a finished portrait but she or he will most likely accommodate your suggestions so as not to damage her or his reputation. If an artist accepts defeat entirely and chooses to add the portrait to her or his store of works for exhibition you must start the commissioning process from scratch and pay the artist's expenses. Bearing in mind the "gentlemanly" nature of the agreement you should also offer part of the fee. Artists belonging to the Royal Society of Portrait Painters ask for a third of their fee in advance and the rest on completion. Finally, does the final bill include framing and varnishing (or casting in the case of a portrait bust)?

The first sitting

The next stage is the first sitting—at home, at work, or in the

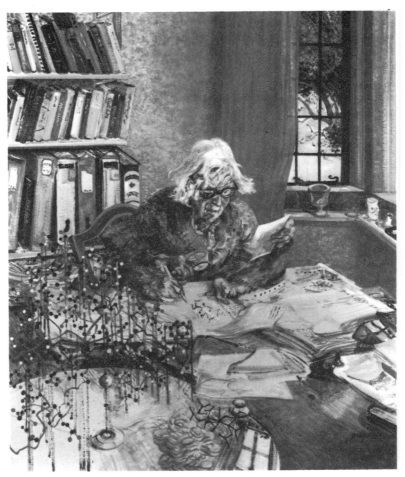

Portrait of Dorothy Hodgkin by Maggi Hembling, 1985

artist's studio—the setting depends on the purpose of the portrait and your choice of iconography. Artists' working methods vary enormously. Some will produce a finished portrait "on the spot" with few sittings. Others will take many photographs, make numerous drawings, and produce the finished work in your absence. Most will produce a study or series of studies at the first sitting. In some cases an artist produces rapid, loosely worked pencil or charcoal drawings as you talk. Others may require total silence and a fixed pose and go for a much more finished piece—even a small watercolour or oil study (or a sculptured maquette). Work produced at this stage gives the subject an opportunity for a useful exchange of views; the artist can tell you how she or he envisages the finished work and you can discuss reservations.

If the first sitting is a success you will be invited to have subsequent sittings and then to view the finished work. Ask your closest friend to give you an honest opinion of the portrait—not just in terms of physical likeness and recognisable iconography but to assess whether the artist has captured your essential character. It should not be too late for amendments to be made or indeed to reject the commission, but you should remember that the purpose of a portrait is not to flatter the vanity of the sitter but to stand as a summation of career or personality or in its own right as a strong and solid work of art.

Think of posterity

If the portrait is not acceptable (for example, to you or the commissioning body) you should say so. It will be almost impossible for you to reject it on artistic grounds—you chose the style, you saw previous work, it is a risk you have to take. What criteria separate a bad painting from a good one, can you argue your case through? There should be fewer problems justifying rejection on the grounds that the portrait is not a true likeness, though sitters are not always the best judges as they never see themselves as others do. If, for example, the commissioning body is really unhappy you should have a "full and frank" discussion with the artist about points you think that she or he has got wrong. Most artists will probably arrange further sittings, make new sketches, and alter or completely repaint the portrait, charging only for additional expenses incurred. On the other hand, if you are presented with a portrait that is a poor likeness but a wonderful work of art, think of posterity. Will it really matter what you looked like? Won't future generations be all the more respectful that you had the foresight to choose such a talented artist?

The task of commissioning a portrait does not end here. The painting will need to be framed and eventually varnished (six months later) or the plaster to be cast, stages that add quite considerably to the cost unless budgeted from the start. Many artists, particularly young unknowns, prefer to frame their work themselves. You should ask to see examples of their framing; it can often be unprofessional and detract from an otherwise good painting. Professional framing is expensive but worth doing. An artist may have a preferred framer, and she or he may wish to visit the framer with you to advise on what is needed—for example, roccoco gilded plasterwork or plain stained wood with canvas slips. Some artists may wish to paint the frame themselves, sometimes extending or "bleeding" elements of the painting on to the frame. Or they may wish it to be carved with motifs reflecting passages in the painting. Whatever the case, you should be sure that you will be happy with the end result. A portrait bust will require a plinth or stand. The artist can advise on your choice: an antique, or a cast of an old style, or something more up to date.

If the portrait is intended for home consumption the story is almost over. Once the finished article has been approved, a nice touch is to invite the artist to a small party at which friends and family can view the portrait and ask about its evolution. If the commission is a formal one it must be presented to the commissioning body, most usually at a private viewing or unveiling. Guests should include the artist, you the sitter, your peer group, the commissioning committee, family and selected friends as well as former and future patrons of the artist. An enthusiastic press officer will ensure that a private viewing becomes a media event and may cajole you and the artist into making a formal statement about the commission. Discuss any misgivings about this kind of circus before it is too late. Check that this stage of the proceedings is covered by a separate entertainment budget as the costs can be quite high. The portrait will need to be displayed and lit for the event. Possibly unveiling will take place away from the portrait's eventual location or for ease of viewing it may be displayed on an easel. It will still need professional lighting and to be hung and relit after the event.

If you have the time, money, and inclination having your por-

---

Factors to consider when planning timescale

- Basic research
- Number and duration of sittings
- Length of time required to complete portrait
- Framing or casting and mounting
- Is the unveiling to take place before or after varnishing?
- Does the artist intend to exhibit it elsewhere afterwards?

---

trait painted can be a challenging and rewarding experience. The more effort you put into it—in terms of adequate preparation and research, facilitating the number and length of sittings required, and being open with the artist—the better the end result. Anything less than total commitment will result in an unsatisfactory commission, and you should think of sitting for a stuio photograph instead.

Useful information

John Player Portrait Award 9 June-3 September 1989. National Portrait Gallery, 2 St Martin's Place, London WC2H oHE (tel 01-930 1552). Open Mon-Sat 10-5, Sun 2-5. Admission free. Catalogue available. Display of 70 outstanding portraits chosen from over 700 entries. All work by artists under the age of 40. Over half the artists exhibited receive commissions from mebers of the public. Commissions can be reasonably priced (hundreds rather than thousands of pounds). Choosing a young unknown can be quite a risk. Alternatively, if you have a fixed idea of the style of portrait you want but haven't the budget to afford the real thing watch out for students who rigidly follow their teachers—a means of acquiring your end at a cost you can afford (not for purists). Further information from the National Portrait Gallery's competitions office.

Royal Society of Portrait Painters Annual Exhibition held in May. The Mall Galleries, The Mall, London SW1 (tel 01-930 6844). Open daily 10-5. Admission free. Open exhibition dominated by work of members of the society. Catalogue includes names and addresses of all members. Huge price range. Further information from the Secretary, Royal Society of Portrait Painters, 17 Carlton House Terrace, London SW1Y 5BG (tel 01-930 6844).

Portrait Centre, New Grafton Gallery, 48 Church Road, Barnes, London SW3 9HH (tel 01-748 8850). Open Tues-Sat 10-5 30. Admission free. Catalogue of artists represented includes brief biographies and lists previous protraits. Examples of work and photographic portfolios held at Gallery. Price range from £4–500 to £4–5000.

Exhibitions concentrating on a single sitter such as the excellent *In Close-up* series in the twentieth century galleries of the National Portrait Gallery are especially useful, including as they do a wide range of media by many diverse artists. In 1986, for example, there was a display on the Nobel Prize winning chemist and crystallographer Professor Dorothy Hodgkin that included portraits by Henry Moore, Graham Sutherland, Bryan Organ, Sheila Fell, and Maggi Hambling and several portrait photographs.

Improve the counselling skills of doctors and nurses in cancer care

PETER MAGUIRE, ANN FAULKNER

The diagnosis and treatment of cancer cause considerable psychological distress and morbidity.[1] But this is resolved in only a minority of patients because those concerned in their care tend to avoid the emotional aspects.[2] They distance themselves for two main reasons. They lack the skills to handle the difficult problems and strong emotions that may emerge if they talk with patients and relatives in any depth. Also, they fear that probing into how a person is adjusting psychologically will do more harm than good.

Fortunately, many doctors and nurses who care for cancer patients realise that their difficulties in communicating with patients and their relatives stem from insufficient training and are eager to remedy this. We describe how to run short intensive workshops to help doctors and nurses improve their skills in interviewing, assessment, and counselling.

Structure

Participants—Nurses often complain that they cannot talk openly with cancer patients because doctors will not let them do so and that doctors ignore important feedback about patients. Doctors usually counter these complaints by stating that nurses are too eager to "pass the buck" to them and do not understand how difficult it is to break bad news and initiate unpleasant treatments. We therefore include both doctors and nurses in the workshops so that these opposing views can be aired, discussed, and resolved. We try to ensure equal representation of hospital and community staff, for the latter tend to excuse their reluctance to talk with cancer patients on the basis that they have still to hear formally from the hospital what patients have been told about their illness and prognosis.

Size—We limit our workshops to 20 people. This ensures that participants are involved fully and have at least one opportunity to practise their skills and be given feedback.

Setting—While workshops can be held in the workplace, it is difficult for participants to avoid being contacted to deal with clinical problems. Nor is there much opportunity for informal sharing of concerns at the end of each day. Consequently, our workshops are residential. We use a centre that has comfortable rooms suitable for both large and small group work and also provides good food and accommodation. This allows participants to devote their attention to the workshops instead of complaints about the setting.

Duration—Three to four days are needed to cover the main agenda and permit discussion about how to apply newly acquired skills while ensuring personal survival.

Teaching

Tutors

The workshops require experienced doctors and nurses to acknowledge that they find certain counselling situations hard to cope with because they lack the relevant skills. They also have to watch demonstration videotapes that show patients and relatives in predicaments. So, strong feelings may be aroused and powerful memories triggered. This requires two experienced tutors (preferably a doctor and a nurse) to monitor reactions and intervene publicly or privately when necessary, which minimises the risk that participants will be harmed and allows potentially damaging situations to be used constructively as in the following example.

While an experienced nurse watched a videotape of an interview between a tutor (PM) and a patient with cancer she became very angry. Her anger seemed out of all proportion, and so the second tutor (AF) asked her if she would explain her reaction. She disclosed that her mother was dying of cancer and suffering terrible pain. She believed her mother was being neglected by the medical staff but felt she could not complain because they were her colleagues. In describing this both she and other participants realised that she was blaming the tutor for other doctors' apparent short-comings.

Methods

It is crucial that teaching methods are congruent with the models of interviewing, assessment, and counselling being taught. So, the beginning of a workshop mirrors the initial phase of an assessment interview with a patient who has requested help. (Key techniques are in parentheses.)

Beginning

We introduce ourselves (self introduction), give the aims of the workshop and the methods we will use (orientation), and check if these are acceptable (negotiation). We add that we are willing to adapt our methods to meet participants' needs (sensitivity to need). Participants are then asked to explain who they are, why they have come, and what they are hoping for (establishing expectations).

They are next asked to think of and disclose problems they have experienced in recent weeks when talking with cancer patients, relatives, and colleagues which they would like to have handled better. They are split into two small groups to do this. Each group appoints a leader who ensures that each participant contributes at least one problem (promoting honest disclosure of key problems). Another member keeps a record of the problems (recording key problems). It is explained that the success of the workshop depends, like counselling, on the level of disclosure. If important problems remain hidden they cannot be discussed and resolved.

When the group reforms a rapporteur from each group describes the problems that have been disclosed. We clarify the nature and extent of each problem by inviting the participants who volunteered the problems to give more detail (clarification, precision). As each problem is clarified it is listed on a flipchart (compiling a problem list). Once all the problems have been mentioned the participants are asked if there are any other problems they would like help with (screening for any other problems).

Agreeing the goals

As in counselling there may be too many problems to cover in the time available. Priorities have to be decided and realistic goals set. Participants are asked in turn to rate how essential it is for them to cover each listed problem on a scale from 0 or no relevance to 10 or most essential. We advise them to think only of their own needs and work situation when giving a rating verbally (disclosing real *v* expected needs). Group scores are calculated for each problem (range 0–200). Problems are then relisted on a flipchart in rank order from the most to least essential.

The agenda of the workshop is decided on the basis of the top eight problems (table I). A problem which produced both very high and very low scores is also included to check the accuracy of participants' self awareness. The problems to be covered are summarised by a tutor and the group asked if this agenda is acceptable (summarise goals, check acceptability). We then explain that the other problems listed will be dealt with briefly in a later session (reviewing unfinished business).

TABLE I—*Problem list*

	Score (maximum = 200)	% of maximum
Breaking bad news	180	90
Patient who has been lied to	178	89
Basic interviewing/assessment	177	88.5
Handling difficult questions	175	87.5
Dealing with the angry patient	171	85.5
Challenging denial	168	84
Sudden, unexpected death	163	81.5
Bereaved relatives	158	79
Breaking collusion	153	76.5
Handling the withdrawn patient	149	74.5

Basic interviewing and assessment

We suggest that participants tackle the least difficult problem first to generate confidence, which is invariably how quickly to establish an empathic relationship with a patient and identify key problems. A videotape showing a tutor conducting an assessment is used to show the aspects to be covered and skills to be used. We expose ourselves to scrutiny to emphasise that we are not perfect interviewers or counsellors and can tolerate constructive feedback.

The aspects covered are history of the patient's illness and treatment to date; patient's perceptions, psychological reactions, and view of the future; and the impact of illness and treatment on the patient's daily life, mood, and key relationships. The following techniques are demonstrated: acknowledging, organising, clarifying, and exploring key verbal and non-verbal cues; how to keep patients to the point and use time optimally but avoid alienation; encouraging precise accounts so that patients make the effort to remember and describe experiences and feelings fully and accurately; and encouraging the expression of feelings.

Key strategies shown are dealing with patients' concerns before professional concerns—like a review of physical systems; ensuring full coverage of one topic before moving to another—for example, the nature and extent of a body image problem before talking about the partner's responses; and obtaining a list of all key problems before giving advice or attempting any resolution. The tapes are stopped at key points and participants invited to suggest which aspects are being covered and why and which techniques and strategies are being used. The interviewing and assessment model is thus made explicit. Once participants have assimilated the model they are split into two groups, each with a tutor, to practise basic interviewing and assessment skills by role play.

Use of role play

Role play allows participants to practise under controlled conditions, and audiotape recording permits playback and discussion. Otherwise much time can be lost in debating whether or not certain skills were used. Most participants are wary of role play because of adverse experiences. We explain, therefore, that we will make it as safe but realistic as possible by observing the following rules: (*a*) Every participant will do a role play. (*b*) The patient, relative, or colleague presenting the problem will be played by the person who volunteered it as a difficult problem in the initial small group discussions. (*c*) A participant should not play a particular role—for example, a bereaved relative—if it is too close to an adverse personal experience (bereavement). (*d*) The role player will not make the problem more difficult than it was in real life. (*e*) The doctor or nurse tackling the problem will be given an explicit, simple but realistic brief. (*f*) Each role player will stay within the brief given. (*g*) If a participant feels stuck in the role play he or she must call time out, otherwise the tutor will do so to avoid embarrassment and humiliation. (*h*) When a role play is stopped the doctor or nurse and the person playing a patient, relative, or colleague will first be asked to comment on how he or she thinks the interaction is going. (*i*) Other members of the group will then be asked to identify strengths in the doctor or nurse's performance. (*j*) Only when they have exhausted all strengths will they be allowed by the tutor to suggest why the doctor or nurse got stuck. (*k*) The group (not the doctor or nurse) will be asked to offer other strategies. (*l*) The doctor or nurse will then be invited to test out these strategies in role play until the problem is resolved.

Briefing

The participant playing the patient, relative, or colleague is taken out of the room and briefed by a tutor who uses the participant's real life experience of the problem to develop the brief. The role player then returns to the room to sit down and "get into role" while the tutor briefs the doctor or nurse. For example: Sheila is a 32 year old housewife who was told two years ago that her breast cancer had been cured by surgery and radiotherapy. She has now developed a recurrence on her scar line and has widespread bony metastases. She has been referred to you as the medical oncologist for advice about further treatment. Your task is to assess her and determine her current problems and whether they are physical, social, or psychological. Remember to signal time out if you feel stuck and I will then ask the group to suggest alternative strategies.

Feedback

The doctor then joins the "patient" and is asked to begin the role play by asking an open question—for example, what problems have brought you here today? The tutor starts the audiotape recording and the role play continues until time out is signalled by the doctor or tutor, usually some three to four minutes later. Each participant in the role play is asked to comment on how it is going, emphasising good points first. The group is then requested to highlight what they liked. Only when no more strengths are forthcoming are constructive criticisms invited by the tutor who asks: Why did the doctor get stuck? The tutor then asks the group to suggest what other strategies might be tried (emphasising a shared approach to problem solving). These strategies are then discussed and tested out in further role play (testing out strategies). The tutor resists offering a solution unless the group fail to resolve the problem (encouraging participants to generate their own solutions). These exercises in role play concerning basic interviewing and assessments are carried out in a 90 minute session (table II).

Problems in counselling

Role play is also used to help participants to learn how to resolve

TABLE II—*Timetable and agenda for workshop*

Day 1:	
3.30 pm	Tea
4.00 pm	Self introduction and orientation
4.30 pm	Identification of problems (small groups)
5.30 pm	Reporting back and negotiating agenda
6.45 pm	Dinner
8.00 pm	Basic interviewing and assessment I
9.00 pm	Close
Day 2:	
9.15 am	Basic interviewing and assessment II (videotape demonstration and discussion)
10.45 am	Coffee
11.15 am	Basic interviewing and assessment (role play)
12.45 pm	Lunch
2.00 pm	Breaking bad news (role play)
3.45 pm	Tea
4.15 pm	Patient advocacy (video)
5.15 pm	Close
Day 3:	
9.15 am	Dealing with anger (role play)
10.15 am	The withdrawn patient (role play)
11.15 am	Dealing with a misinformed patient (role play)
12.45 pm	Lunch
2.15 pm	Sudden unexpected death (role play)
	Challenging denial (role play)
3.45 pm	Tea
4.15 pm	Breaking collusion (video)
5.15 pm	Close
Day 4:	
9.15 am	Breaking collusion (video) continued
10.00 am	Unfinished business (discussion)
10.45 am	Coffee
11.15 am	Survival (discussion)
12.45 pm	Lunch
1.45 pm	Evaluation
3.00 pm	Close

other problems on the main agenda, such as "how to break bad news" and "relate to an angry patient." Explicit briefs are given based on real life situations disclosed by the participants.

For example, John had a lymphoma diagnosed two years ago and was treated with chemotherapy and radiotherapy. He experienced severe adverse effects, particularly conditioned vomiting. He nearly opted out but was persuaded to continue by the argument that he had a 95% chance of a complete cure. His lymphoma has returned and further chemotherapy has been suggested. He feels very angry and is refusing treatment.

John is then played by the doctor who encountered this predicament. This gives the doctor valuable insight into what it might have been like to be on the receiving end of care.

These problems are covered in subsequent sessions (table II), and these sessions, like counselling, can be intense and emotionally draining but enriching. They are separated by long coffee and lunch breaks (need for time out) and further videotape demonstrations which are both serious and humorous (need for light relief). The role playing is distributed equitably within each group so that no one takes an undue burden (sharing the load).

Ending

Unfinished business—After completion of the agreed goals unfinished business is reviewed.

Survival—Participants are invited to discuss the methods they use to ensure that they cope when confronted by the emotional demands of caring for cancer patients. They also consider how they might cope if they relinquish their distancing tactics and apply their new skills when they return to their place of work. The importance of sharing concerns promptly with colleagues, whether formally in support groups or informally, is emphasised.

Review—Participants are asked to say what they found most and least helpful in the workshop (asking for feedback) and to suggest improvements (demonstrate willingness to learn).

Follow up—A one and a half day workshop is held six months later to discuss how far participants have been able to apply what they learnt and obtain adequate support. It also allows them to discuss if their new skills were effective (validation) and to practise more difficult counselling tasks.

Discussion

We are attempting to meet an important need for training in counselling skills. An analysis of audiotapes of the role playing in the initial workshops has confirmed that this need is real and substantial. But we continue to be impressed by the willingness of experienced doctors and nurses to subject themselves to such close scrutiny. For it is hard for experienced doctors and nurses to admit to being inadequate. Fortunately, the feedback from participants has been consistently positive with most participants claiming that they have improved their skills and become more confident about assessing and counselling cancer patients.

The follow up workshops also suggest that these improvements are maintained, but we have started on an objective study to determine if these claims of short and longer term improvement are confirmed by independent assessment.

References

1   Greer S. Cancer: psychiatric aspects. In: Granville-Grossman K, ed. *Recent advances in clinical psychiatry*. London: Churchill Livingstone, 1985; 87–103.
2   Maguire P. Barriers to psychological care of the dying. *Br Med J* 1985; **291**: 1711–13.

Communicate with cancer patients: 1 Handling bad news and difficult questions

PETER MAGUIRE, ANN FAULKNER

We suggest how to handle situations in communicating with patients with cancer which doctors and nurses commonly find difficult.[1]

Breaking bad news

It is important to accept that you cannot soften the impact of bad news since it is still bad news however it is broken. The key to breaking it is to try to slow down the speed of the transition from a patient's perception of himself as being well to a realisation that he (or she) has a life threatening disease. If you break the news too abruptly it will disorganise him psychologically and he will have difficulty adapting. Alternatively, it may provoke denial because the news is too painful to assimilate. Thus you should avoid stating baldly, "I am afraid you've got cancer," and instead warn him that you are about to communicate serious information by saying, for example, "I am afraid it looks more serious than an ulcer."

While you may be tempted to soften this immediately by adding: "Even so we should still be able to do something about it," resist this and pause to let your warning sink in. This will also allow you time to monitor how your patient is reacting. What you say next depends on his response. A question like: "What do you mean not just an ulcer?" suggests that he wants more information. If, however, he says, "That's all right doctor I'll leave it up to you," he is suggesting that he does not wish to learn more at this time. By using a hierarchy of euphemisms for the word cancer, such as a few odd cells, a kind of tumour, a bit cancerous, it is possible to manage the transition so that you can establish how far your patient wants to go at each stage.

Doctor: I'm afraid it's more than just an ulcer. . . .
Mr K: What do you mean more than just an ulcer?
Doctor: Some of the cells looked abnormal under the microscope. . . .
Mr K: Abnormal?
Doctor: They looked cancerous.
Mr K: You mean I've got cancer?
Doctor: I am afraid so, yes.

You should next explore how he feels about this information and why. This will usually reveal that there are good reasons for his responses.

Doctor: How does this news leave you feeling?
Mr K: Terrified! I've always had this thing about cancer. I've always been frightened of getting it. Two of my uncles died of it. They both had a bad time. Suffered terrible pain and wasted away . . . to nothing.
Doctor: So you're frightened you're going to go the same way.
Mr K: I'm bound to be scared, aren't I?
Doctor: Yes, you are in view of those experiences. It must be hard for you. Any other reasons you are terrified?
Mr K: I hate being a burden. My wife has enough to contend with.

Sometimes a patient's responses are better signalled by nonverbal behaviour. It then helps if you acknowledge this and invite him to discuss his feelings.

Doctor: I'm sorry I've had to give you this news. I can see you're distressed. Would you like to talk about it?
Mr C: It is so incredibly unfair. I have always been careful with what I eat. I've not been a drinker. I have exercised regularly. To get cancer now, just when we're getting on our feet as a family, seems so unfair. It makes me feel very bitter.

Having established his immediate responses you should establish any other concerns before attempting to give information about the treatment you propose and the likely outcome. Otherwise he will remain preoccupied with these concerns, will not heed your advice, and may misperceive what you say.

Doctor: We have explored why you feel so terrified at knowing you have cancer. Has it caused you to have any other worries?
Mr C: Yes.
Doctor: Would you like to tell me about them?
Mr C: I'm not sure whether I should go ahead with my plan to move house.
Doctor: Sounds as though you're worried that we may not be able to do anything for your cancer.
Mr C: Yes I am.
Doctor: I'll come back to that in a minute. Before I do, do you have any other concerns?
Mr C: Yes. Who will look after the children if I don't make it?
Doctor: So, you are concerned about whether or not to move house, about your children.
Mr C: Yes I am.
Doctor: Anything else you're concerned about?
Mr C: No.
Doctor: Are you sure?
Mr C: Yes.

Once you have established your patient's concerns you should be able to decide if they can be resolved. It is important that your statements about these concerns are realistic but maintain hope.

Mrs H: It is the prospect of pain that terrifies me.
Doctor: I can understand that.
Mrs H: Can you do anything?
Doctor: There is every chance that we can. So it is very important you let me know if you have any pain, and we can see what we can do.

Similarly, efforts to foster and maintain hope about the outcome of treatment should be appropriate.

Doctor: When we removed your cancer we found that a few of the nodes under your arm were affected and removed those as well. To be sure we mop up all the cancer we ought to give you some chemotherapy. There is then a good chance you'll be OK.
Mrs M: You're not certain?

Doctor: No I can't be certain, but I do think there's every chance of a reasonable outcome in your case providing you have some chemotherapy.

When the prognosis is poor the doctor can usually indicate that something can be done.

Doctor: You're right, you have got lung cancer.

Mr S: That's what I thought. I keep coughing up blood and I've lost so much weight. Are you going to be able to do anything about it?

Doctor: Yes, I think so. I'm hopeful that we'll get some response with radiotherapy and that you will feel much less ill.

Mr S: Only some response?

Doctor: While we should be able to shrink it considerably, I'm not certain we'll be able to get it all.

Mr S: You mean some could be left?

Doctor: There could be. But we would then consider giving you a course of strong drugs. I think we ought to start with radiotherapy first. I'm pretty certain we can get it under control and that will make you feel better.

Mr S: I suppose I have to be grateful for that.

Doctor: I can understand that you are disappointed that I can't guarantee getting rid of it all, but I think it likely you'll feel better once you start radiotherapy. Then maybe you won't be so worried. We will still have the drugs at our disposal should they be necessary.

Even when you cannot eradicate the disease it is still important to explore your patient's feelings and concerns since it is likely that you can still do something.

General practitioner: You remember that you came to see me because you were feeling so weak and were worried your cancer had come back and was spreading . . . and I sent you to the hospital for tests?

Mr F: Yes I do.

General practitioner: Good. The reason I came round this morning is to give you the results of those tests they did at the hospital.

Mr F: Yes, I guessed that. What did they find?

General practitioner: I am afraid your guess was right, the

cancer has come back. That's the reason why you've been feeling so weak and tired.

Mr F: I thought so. Are you going to be able to do anything for me?

General practitioner: I'm afraid I do not feel that further treatment is going to make much difference to the cancer.

The general practitioner then explored Mr F's resulting concerns and an important issue emerged. He was worried that he might suffer severe pain.

General practitioner: I'm sorry to have to tell you this. It can't be easy for you. Do you have any particular worries?

Mr F: I'm terrified of getting bad pain.

General practitioner: If that happens I hope we will be able to control your pain with strong pain killers. Let me know if you're having any problems with pain, or any other symptoms, come to that. The sooner we know about it the sooner we should be able to do something.

Mr F: Yes I can see that.

General practitioner: Apart from getting pain, are there any other concerns?

Mr F: No.

General practitioner: I'm sorry it's worked out this way, but we certainly should be able to do something to help you if there are any problems with pain. It's very important we keep in close touch.

The doctor did not say that he could eliminate any pain, for this would be false reassurance. Instead, he indicated that there was every chance he could palliate the pain. He also showed that he was prepared to discuss other concerns.

This tragedy of moving from acknowledging and exploring the nature and basis of any strong feelings to identifying key concerns is essential if the breaking of bad news is to be managed effectively. It allows the patient to be "lifted" from being overwhelmed to feeling hopeful that something can be done.

Handling difficult questions

Many doctors and nurses fear that if they get into a dialogue with patients with cancer they will be asked difficult questions—

for example, Is it cancer?[2] When such a question is asked it is difficult to know what response is wanted by the patient. Does he (or
she) want the reassurance that it isn't cancer (because he wants to
deny the reality of his illness) or the truth? Only the patient can
suggest the direction he wishes to follow. You can usually discover
this by saying, "I would be happy to answer your question" and
then reflecting his question back to him by asking, "But what
makes you ask that question?" You should then explore if there are
other reasons why he asked it. It will then become clear if the
patient is asking the question because he has guessed what is going
on and wants confirmation that he is right.

Mr M: Is it cancer?
Specialist nurse: I would be happy to answer your question, but
can I first ask you why you're asking me?
Mr M: It's obvious isn't it?
Specialist nurse: Why obvious?
Mr M: I have lost two stones in weight, I'm feeling weaker day
by day and still coughing up blood. It's got to be cancer.
Specialist nurse: Any other reasons why you are so sure that
you've got cancer?
Mr M: I've been a heavy smoker all my life. The doctors want to
give me radiotherapy. You only get radiotherapy for one thing and
that's cancer.
Specialist nurse: Yes, I'm afraid you're right.
Mr M: I knew it, I'm not a fool. Why did they tell me they were
just giving me radiotherapy as an insurance?
Specialist nurse: I honestly don't know. But look, would you like
to talk more about it?
Mr M: Yes I would. What I really want to know—is radiotherapy going to make any difference?
Specialist nurse: We're hopeful that it will get the cancer under
control and that some of the symptoms you're complaining about
will improve considerably.
Mr M: That sounds better than I thought, I thought I was a
goner.
Specialist nurse: A goner?
Mr M: I thought I'd only a few days to live at most.
Specialist nurse: That's not the case. There is a real prospect
that the treatment will help you feel better and keep you going for
some time.

Some patients indicate that they wish to deny what is happening.

Mrs R: I'm going to get better aren't I?

Medical oncologist: What makes you ask that?

Mrs R: You and your team tell me that I have some kind of lymphoma. I can't accept that. I'm certain it is an infection I picked up when I was out in the tropics.

Medical oncologist: I don't want to argue with you about that. The key thing is that you continue with our treatment.

Mrs R: I'm happy to do that.

Conclusion

You may have noticed that the strategies we advise are determined by the patient's responses and not decided unilaterally by the doctor or nurse. We do not expect you to accept them unquestioningly but hope that you will try them out with patients in your care.

References

1   Maguire P, Faulkner A. How to do it: improve the counselling skills of doctors and nurses in cancer care. *Br Med J* 1988; **297**: 847–9.
2   Maguire P. Barriers to psychological care of the dying. *Br Med J* 1985; **291**: 1711–13.

Communicate with cancer patients: 2 Handling uncertainty, collusion, and denial

PETER MAGUIRE, ANN FAULKNER

Breaking bad news often prompts patients to ask questions about their future like: How long have I got? You then have to help them cope with uncertainty without them becoming demoralised.

Handling uncertainty

When asked: How long have I got? it is tempting to give a finite (Oh, three months) or range (Anything from a month to six months) of time. But such predictions are usually inaccurate, tend to err on the optimistic side, and cause problems for patients and their families. Patients then pace themselves according to the time they believe is left. If they deteriorate earlier than expected and are prevented from achieving planned goals they will feel cheated and bitter. Relatives can find an unexpectedly prolonged survival ("borrowed time") hard to cope with because they have used up their physical and emotional resources. So it is better to acknowledge your uncertainty and the difficulties that this will cause.

Doctor: You asked me how long he has. The trouble is, I don't know. I realise this uncertainty must be difficult for you.

Mrs W: It is. It is terrible knowing that he is going to die but not knowing when. I mean it could be in one month's time or next Christmas.

Doctor: That's the trouble, I just don't know how long it will be.

You should next check if she would like to know the signs and symptoms that would herald further deterioration.

Doctor: What I can do, but only if you would like me to, is tell you what changes would suggest he is beginning to deteriorate further.
Mrs W: Yes, I think that would help me.
Doctor: He will probably complain of feeling breathless, weak, and start going off his food.

You can then encourage her to try to use the intervening time.

Doctor: But as long as there are no signs like that I think you can take it that he is relatively OK. So, you should try to make the most of this time if you can. Is there anything you would particularly like to do?

Later, add that you are prepared to check him regularly, and show a willingness to negotiate the frequency of such check ups.

Doctor: I think it would help if I saw him from time to time to monitor how he is doing. How often would you like me to do that?
Mrs W: Would every month be OK?
Doctor: Yes, fine.

You should explain that if anything unforeseen occurs between these assessments you should be contacted immediately. This gives patients and relatives confidence that they have a "life line."

Doctor: If you are worried at any stage between his appointments you must get in touch with me. I can then assess him and decide what needs to be done.

Few patients or relatives abuse this offer.
When some patients or relatives face uncertainty they show that they do not want any markers.

Doctor: Would you like me to tell you how you might recognise if Peter's health is deteriorating?
Mrs B: No, I'll leave it to you. You're the expert.

Sometimes the uncertainty concerns issues other than "how long." Again you should acknowledge the uncertainty and establish any resulting worries.

Doctor: I sense that this uncertainty is a major problem for you.

Mr J: It is. I feel helpless not knowing what's going to happen or how it's going to happen.

Doctor: What are you worried about in particular?

Mr J: I'm worried about how I'm going to die. I don't want to be a burden on my family, and I'm not sure what to expect after death.

Doctor: Any other concerns?

Mr J: Isn't that enough?

Doctor: Yes, it is, but I just want to make sure I establish all your concerns before we discuss them in detail.

By separating out and exploring each concern the patient begins to see that there is some prospect that they can be tackled.

Breaking collusion

It is commonly alleged that relatives withhold the truth because they cannot face the pain of what is happening and wish to deny it. More commonly, however, it is an act of love. They cannot bear to cause anguish to their loved one. Approaching collusion from this perspective makes it possible to respect relatives' reasons and work positively with them. The first step is to acknowledge the collusion and then explore and validate the reasons for it.

Doctor: You've told me that you don't feel Richard ought to know what is going on. Why do you feel that?

Mrs P: I'm terrified that if he's told he'll simply fall apart. I wouldn't want that, I couldn't bear it.

Doctor: Well you know him best and you could be right. It could be that if he's told he will fall apart. Have you any other reasons why you feel he shouldn't be told?

Mrs P: I think he'd just give up and turn his face to the wall.

Doctor: Any other reasons?

Mrs P: No.

Doctor: So you have good reason for him not being told.

Mrs P: Yes.

It is then important to establish the emotional cost of the collusion.

Doctor: I now understand why you have kept the information from him, but what effect has this been having on you?

Mrs P: It's been a terrible strain. I'm feeling extremely tense, I'm not sleeping as well as I should, I'm getting nightmares.

Doctor: Would you like to tell me about your nightmares?

Mrs P: He seems to be getting smaller and smaller, he seems to be wasting away.

Doctor: That's, I suppose, what could happen, isn't it, given that he is dying?

Mrs P: (In tears) Yes it is and I'm very worried about it.

Doctor: So it sounds as if you are finding it a strain!

Mrs P: It is. It's a big strain. I worry that he will begin to guess. He's already commented that I seem quieter than usual.

Doctor: Just how tense have you been?

Mrs P: At times I feel at screaming point and I'm taking it out on the children. I feel bad about that, but I just can't see how I can tell him without him falling apart.

Doctor: Are you experiencing any other problems because of not telling him?

Mrs P: Yes, we're not talking together like we used to. I'd like to be extra loving to him, but if I am he'll guess. He says I'm backing off. But I can't explain to him why. It's horrible. Just when I want to be close to him a barrier is growing between us.

Doctor: So, there are two good reasons for trying to consider whether there's some way round this, the strain on you and the effect on your relationship with your husband.

Mrs P: Yes.

Doctor: So would you like me to suggest how we might be able to do something about it?

Mrs P: But you're not going to tell him are you?

Doctor: No, what I'm going to discuss doesn't involve telling him, would you like me to go into it?

Mrs P: Yes, I would.

You should now indicate that you would like to chat with her partner to check whether he has any idea of what is happening to him. You should reinforce that you have no intention of telling him and enter into a contract to this effect.

Doctor: Let me emphasise that I have no intention of telling him. What I'd like to do is to chat to him to see what he's thinking about the present situation. It may be that he will reveal that he knows he has cancer. If that's the case there will be no reason to maintain the pretence.

Mrs P: But you're not going to tell him are you?

Doctor: No I'm not, I will simply check whether he knows. If your hunch that he doesn't have any idea is correct, that's the end of the matter. I won't say anything.

Mrs P: (Reluctantly) All right then.

Your next task is to establish her partner's level of awareness. You should ask an appropriate directive question which elicits his view of what is happening and then explore the cues he gives.

Doctor: I wanted to have a chat to see how you feel things are going.

Mr P: Not very well.

Doctor: Not very well?

Mr P: Isn't it obvious? I'm not having any more treatment. The hospital don't want to see me again but I'm still getting the pain. I'm losing weight and I haven't much energy. I'm in bed all the time now.

Doctor: So what are you making of this?

Mr P: I think it's the end, isn't it?

Doctor: Are there any other reasons why you're beginning to feel it's the end?

Mr P: I've always known that what they've told me was a pre-cancerous ulcer was a cancer. Now what's happening is confirming that I was right. I'm lying here just wondering why no one has levelled with me.

Doctor: It sounds as though you've known for some time what's happening.

Mr P: Yes, I have, but I didn't want to upset my wife. She has enough on her plate with me being ill, and having to run around all the time.

You now should confirm that he is right ("I'm afraid you are right") and then seek permission to convey his awareness to his wife, indicating that she knows the diagnosis. Then negotiate with the couple to see if they are prepared to talk with you to establish their concerns.

As you help the couple talk you may notice that the patient is angry with you. This usually indicates that he feels talking is a waste of time because it will not change the outcome of his disease. If you get this feeling acknowledge it.

Doctor: Would you like to say how this leaves you feeling?

Mr P: What's the point? It's not going to be of much use.

Doctor: It sounds as if you might be feeling that it's no use because it won't make any difference to your situation.

Mr P: That's right; it's not going to stop me dying is it?

Doctor: No you're absolutely right. That's the one thing I can't do and I'm sorry about that. But it may help if we talk about how you're feeling and what you're worried about. It is quite likely there is something I can do to help you both. However, I will understand if you decide not to talk to me.

Mr P: I suppose I've nothing to lose by talking.

Breaking collusion is painful for the doctor because he witnesses the love between a couple and the effects of imminent loss. But it is important to break it as soon as it becomes a problem. Otherwise important unfinished business will be left unresolved. The patient is then likely to be distressed and may become morbidly anxious and depressed. This mental suffering will lower the threshold at which the patient experiences physical symptoms like pain and sickness and cause problems with symptom relief. Failing to deal with important practical and emotional unfinished business also makes it difficult for relatives to resolve their grief.

Challenging denial

Patients use denial when the truth is too painful to bear. So denial should not be challenged unless it is creating serious problems for the patient or relative. In challenging denial it is important to do it gently so that fragile defences are not disrupted but firmly enough so that any awareness can be explored and developed.

It is first worth asking the patient to give an account of what has happened since his (or her) illness was first discovered and explore how he felt at each key point—for example, when he first developed the symptoms, saw a specialist, was investigated, and was told about his illness. He can then explain what he perceives is wrong, and thus may provide glimpses of doubt: "I'm certain it's an ulcer, at least I'm pretty sure it is." By repeating "Pretty sure?" you may prompt him to say, "Well I suppose there could be some doubt." The cue "some doubt" can next be explored to see if he owns up to the possibility that the ulcer could be cancer. It is then important to interpret what is happening by saying, "Part of you prefers to believe that it's an ulcer, but another part of you is willing to consider that it is more serious." The patient can then retreat to denial or develop his awareness further ("I've been trying to kid myself that it's an ulcer, but deep down I realise it's cancer").

If this strategy fails look for and challenge any inconsistencies between the patient's experiences and perceptions.

Doctor: You say you were far bigger in this pregnancy than in your two previous ones. Did you consider why that might be?

Mrs J: I thought it was just one of those things. I didn't think anything more about it.

Doctor: Are you sure?

Mrs J: Yes I am sure it was a normal pregnancy. The reason I'm still feeling so weak is because I didn't take it too well.

The patient had developed ovarian cancer which was so advanced that little treatment could be offered. She preferred to deny this and insisted that her symptoms represented normal sequelae of pregnancy.

If challenging inconsistencies fails to dent denial check if there is "a window." Do this by asking: "I can understand that you feel it is an infection. But is there any time, even a moment, when you consider that it may not be so simple?" The patient may say "No," in which case you have to accept that the patient finds it too painful to look at what is happening. Alternatively, the patient may admit "Yes, there is. Sometimes I feel it could be something much more sinister." Exploring what the patient means by "sinister" may help him acknowledge that he has something much more serious than an ulcer. This then helps him shift from denial into relative or full awareness of his illness or prognosis.

He may then oscillate between denial and awareness. So, do not assume what stance he is going to take but explore it each time by asking: How do you feel things are going?

Conclusion

The best way to validate our guidelines is to try them out in practice. Either they will work and promote confidence or they will prompt you to develop other strategies.